Essential
PRANAYAMA

Essential
PRANAYAMA

Breathing Techniques for Balance, Healing, and Peace

JERRY GIVENS

ROCKRIDGE
PRESS

For general information on our other products and services or to obtain technical support, please contact our Customer Care Department within the United States at (866) 744-2665, or outside the United States at (510) 253-0500.

Rockridge Press publishes its books in a variety of electronic and print formats. Some content that appears in print may not be available in electronic books, and vice versa.

Interior and Cover Designer: Patricia Fabricant
Art Producer: Sue Smith
Editor: John Makowski
Production Editor: Ruth Sakata Corley
Illustrations © 2020 Christian Dellavedova/AAARep.net.
Patterns © Creative Market; © Shutterstock.

ISBN: 978-1-64611-739-0 | eBook 978-1-64611-740-6
R0

To all of my students,
who continue to inspire me in
their dedication and growth

Contents

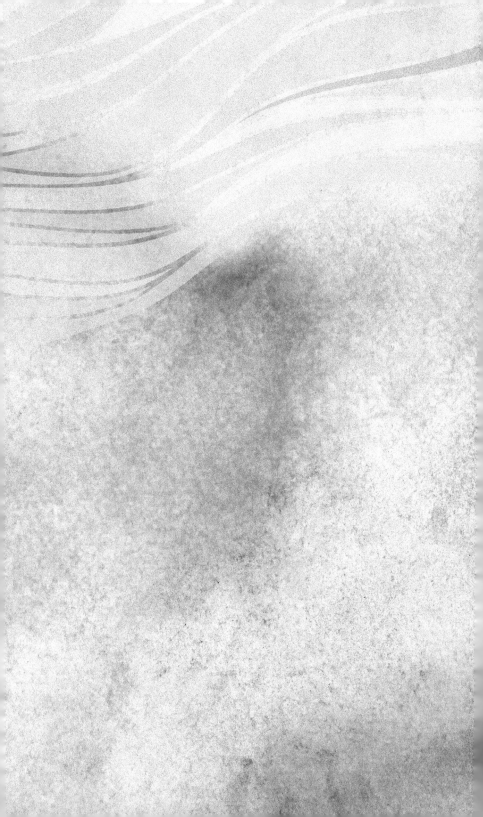

Introduction

I fell into the practice of yoga purely by chance. As a college sophomore, I worked a full-time labor-intensive job and had a full course load. I was stressed out and burned out, trying to balance work, school, homework, and a small semblance of a social life. Little did I know that when I stepped into my first yoga class on a snowy January night in 2006 (with a coupon for a free class), I was starting on a journey that would culminate in thousands of hours of formal training, various assistantships, tens of thousands of hours spent teaching people of all ages and backgrounds, adventures teaching around the world, and now the compilation of teachings of *pranayama* in this book.

Pranayama is a key aspect of the teachings of yoga, and I use these techniques on a daily basis, both in my personal practice and in my teachings. I continue to personally reap the benefits of these practices, and I see my students flourish with their use as well. Many people enter into their yoga practice understanding only its physical benefits. They want to be flexible. They want to stand on their heads. They want to be toned. What they find as they deepen into their practice is that through the manipulation of their breath, the physical benefits are enhanced, along with a vast array of energetic, psychological, and spiritual benefits that they might not have expected. All of a sudden, they find that they are calmer in postures, they are less reactive to stress, and they are more emotionally and psychologically resilient.

Since 2008, I have been leading students and seekers through these pranayama techniques and helping them build lifestyles that improve their overall well-being. When I first started teaching, my main audience was college students (a life from which I had just recently graduated). Like me in college, many of my students were overwhelmed, anxious, uncertain, fearful, and looking for answers on how to "be" in the world. They wanted to suffer less. They came to me seeking to regulate the restless fluctuations of their lives and minds. They needed to learn how to calm down when they were stressed or anxious. They needed to know how to get more energy when they were lethargic, depressed, or burning out. With many of the techniques in this book, they built resiliency and learned to regulate themselves to become calmer, more vital, and overall healthier.

My hope for you, dear reader, is the same as it is for all of the students that I have had the pleasure of teaching. I would like you to learn pranayama, add it to your wellness tool belt, and incorporate these ancient breathing techniques into your daily life. Let these practices empower you to shift your energetic state and to find balance within yourself.

How to Use This Book

This handy and easy-to-use book will take you on a journey through the spectrum of pranayama, from its rich history to techniques and sequences for practitioners of all levels (beginner, intermediate, and advanced). In chapter 1, we'll discuss where these techniques came from, their energetic principles, the benefits of these practices, and what you'll need to be successful moving forward. In chapter 2, we will cover the building blocks of pranayama, including the different ways to breathe and which postures will be best for you. Chapters 3 through 5 will cover 45 pranayama techniques, ranging in practice level, with lots of tips and tricks. These practice chapters have detailed instructions for practitioners of all levels, from those who are new to pranayama to those with a seasoned practice. Lastly, in chapter 6, we will get creative and combine various techniques from the previous three chapters into sequences, helping you enhance the effects of the techniques and take your pranayama practice to the next level. We'll even discuss how you can make your own unique sequences to best suit your individual practice.

It is with great pleasure that I pass these teachings along to you. Take your time, be patient with yourself, and, most of all, just breathe.

Namaste,
Jerry Givens

one

ALL ABOUT PRANAYAMA

The breath is a fascinating function of human life. Without trying, we breathe as we sleep, work, and live, but there is more to breathing than just staying alive. In fact, through the breathing practices of pranayama, you can improve your overall wellness. In this first chapter, I'll introduce the history of these techniques, their general functions, and how they work to help your nervous system, body, and mind. You don't have to be an expert to practice pranayama, as I'll describe techniques that are perfect for beginners and advanced practitioners alike, including some tips to help you at each stage along the way.

WHAT IS PRANAYAMA?

Pranayama is more than just "breath work," as it is commonly misinterpreted. It is a series of techniques through which life force energy is stimulated, expanded, and balanced with the systematic controlling of the breath. These techniques can range from smaller practices, such as witnessing the breath, to more complex exercises that take time and repetition to master. These techniques are done seated, lying down, or in specific postures, as described throughout this book.

The word *pranayama* is a conjunction of the two Sanskrit words *prana* and *ayama*. *Prana* refers to the animating life force energy within all things, similar to *qi* (*chi*) in Buddhism. When prana is rich in supply, your system is energized, and you are balanced psychologically. *Ayama* is a verb that means to "stretch" or "extend" in reference to the action of prana. Literally translated, *pranayama* means to "extend life force energy" to make you more vital, clear-minded, and energized.

Many traditions include pranayama in their wellness practices, including Buddhism, Hinduism, and, of course, yoga. Historically, pranayama is the fourth "limb" of *raja yoga*, described by the sage Patanjali prior to 400 CE in the *Yoga Sutras* as an accompaniment to yoga *asanas* (postures) and a preparatory step for deep states of meditation. Though it has been a part of classical yoga for millennia, many yoga classes taught today in the West omit pranayama or misunderstand its usage. When combined intelligently with certain yoga postures and flows, the effects of pranayama can be amplified, and your experience in postures can be deepened.

A CLOSER LOOK AT PRANA

Prana is understood as life force energy, the sense of being that animates and moves you. At its essence, it is vitality. When prana in the body is low, you can feel sluggish, stuck, or even ill. According to the *The Hatha Yoga Pradipika*, a 15th-century Sanskrit manual on *hatha yoga* by Svatmarama, there are five main movements of prana in your body, called *vayus*, or "wind," that govern your overall system, including digestion, circulation, and elimination. Sometimes these movements can be lacking when there is not enough prana in your body. Through pranayama practices, you can increase the prana in your body and dictate the movements of energy that need more pranic support.

The Five Prana Vayus

1. Udana Vayu – The upward and outward movement of energy. This vayu governs enthusiasm, inspiration, expansion, and ascension. As prana enters the body, *udana* moves it upward toward the throat and face. With pranayama, *udana vayu* is affected by controlling the inhalation side of the breath and any retention of the breath after inhalation.

2. Prana Vayu – (Sometimes called "Pran" Vayu): The inward and upward movement of energy. This vayu governs the intake of prana into the body, as well as inhalation, eating, drinking, sensory impression, and mental experiences, and it is energizing and vitalizing. *Prana vayu* controls prana as it enters the body through the region of the chest and then ascends. With pranayama, prana vayu is affected by controlling the inhalation side of the breath and its capacity in the body.

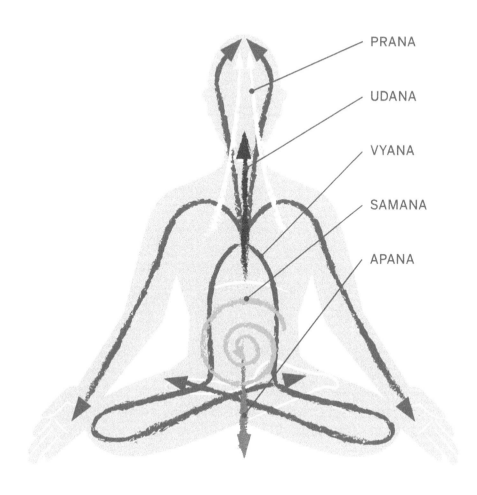

PRANA

UDANA

VYANA

SAMANA

APANA

3. **Samana Vayu** – The assimilating, inward-spiraling movement of energy. This vayu governs the assimilation of food, oxygen, and all experiences into the system. As prana enters the body, *samana* spirals it inward to coalesce around the navel center. With pranayama, *samana vayu* is affected by balancing the lengths and capacity of both the inhalation and exhalation.

4. **Apana Vayu** – The downward and outward movement of energy. This vayu governs the elimination of waste, as well as exhalation, energetic grounding, childbirth, and the removal of negative emotional and psychological experiences. *Apana vayu* moves prana downward toward the reproductive organs and out of the body, aiding with letting go. With pranayama, apana vayu is affected by controlling the exhalation side of the breath.

5. **Vyana Vayu** – The expanding and circulating movement of energy. This vayu governs the circulation of nutrients in the blood and bodily fluids, emotions and thoughts, and engagement in the wider world. *Vyana vayu* spirals from the center of the body and expands outward, integrating prana into the body and world. With pranayama, vyana vayu is affected by controlling the capacity of both the inhalation and exhalation.

Brahmana, Langhana, and Sama Vritti Energetic Effects

There are three energetic effects in yoga: *brahmana*, *langhana*, and *sama vritti*, which can be influenced by meditation, asana (yoga postures), and pranayama.

1. **Brahmana (Expansion)** – The energetic effect of increased energy, vitality building, and extroverted energy. With brahmana pranayama, you can move static energy and excite the nervous system into action. Quicker and more energetic breathing rhythms, full breaths in the chest and ribs, and focus on the inhalation will induce brahmana. You might consider brahmana practices earlier in the day or when you're feeling lethargic, foggy, drained, or depressed.

2. **Langhana (Reduction)** – The energetic effect of calm, grounding, and introverted energy. Through langhana pranayama, you can reduce excess frenetic energy and calm the nervous system. Slower breathing rhythms, breath in the belly, and focus on the exhalation will stimulate langhana. Times when you might consider a langhana practice include during the evening as you prepare for sleep, while experiencing insomnia or overstimulation, after significant trauma, or while feeling general restlessness in your body and mind.

3. **Sama Vritti (Balance)** – The energetic effect of balance. Sama vritti pranayama uses a balance of both brahmana and langhana effects to bring the system into balance. Evening out the length and capacity of the breath on both the inhalation and exhalation, including any holding of the breath, will create a sama vritti effect. If you're not sure what kind of practice you need energetically, sama vritti practices are the perfect solution.

Pranayama is meant to be used in tandem with other types of wellness and health systems, including conventional medicine, and is not intended or instructed to be a substitute. The information shared here is not meant to diagnose or suggest treatment for any health-related concerns. Always consult with your physician regarding any medical issues you may have.

HOW THE BODY BREATHES

Breathing is a result of the combined effort of the respiratory system involving many organs working together simultaneously. As you inhale, the diaphragm drops, the rib cage moves outward, and air rushes into the vacuum created. As you exhale, the diaphragm relaxes, the rib cage contracts, and the air is pushed out. The primary function of the respiratory system is the exchange of oxygen and carbon dioxide in your body. By changing or controlling the breath with pranayama, you can adjust the balances of oxygen and carbon dioxide.

Here's a quick overview of the organs of the respiratory system and how they function during the breathing process:

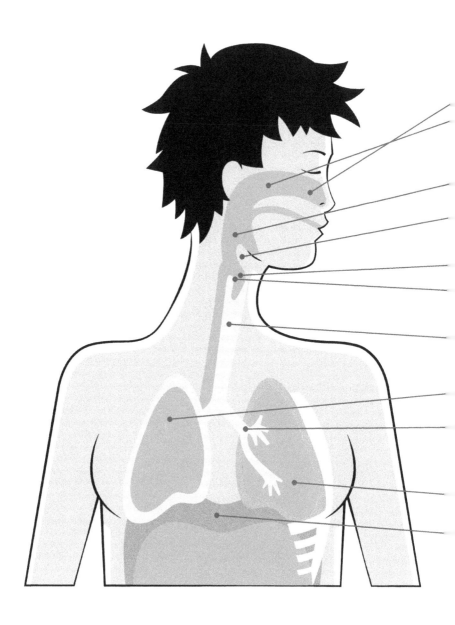

NOSE/MOUTH — The nose and mouth are the passageways for air coming into and out of the body.

TURBINATES — Turbinates are small bony structures, surrounded by a mucous membrane inside of the nasal cavities, that help humidify, warm, and filter the air by removing pollutants before the air is processed by the rest of the respiratory system.

PHARYNX — Also known as the throat, the pharynx is the passageway for food and air.

EPIGLOTTIS — The epiglottis is a small flap at the base of your throat that covers the larynx when swallowing, making sure food and drinks don't go "down the wrong pipe."

LARYNX — Also known as the vocal cords, the larynx is located just below the epiglottis.

GLOTTIS — The glottis is a part of the vocal cords that expands and contracts when you breathe and speak to alter airflow and sound.

TRACHEA — The trachea is the main airway from the throat to the lungs and is commonly referred to as the "windpipe."

LUNGS — The lungs are organs that absorb oxygen as you inhale and release carbon dioxide as you exhale.

BRONCHI & BRONCHIOLES — As air enters the lungs, it moves from the trachea into branching airways, or the left and right bronchus tubes. As the bronchi get smaller farther into the lungs, they are then considered bronchioles.

ALVEOLI — Once the air moves through the bronchioles, it enters the alveoli, small air sacs where oxygen and carbon dioxide are exchanged.

DIAPHRAGM — The diaphragm is your primary breathing muscle, an umbrella-shaped muscle beneath your lungs and heart that initiates and perpetuates the breathing process.

THE ENERGY BODY

In yogic philosophy and psychology, prana flows through the body via energy channels called *nadis*, which pass the prana through tiny spinning vortices of energy and mind called *chakras*. Pranayama, using the logic of the vayus, helps regulate and control the movement of prana through the nadis and brings prana to the chakras in need.

The Nadis

Within the body, there are thousands of fine, wirelike structures called nadis that conduct prana similar to how your blood vessels and veins carry blood throughout your body. Just like how waste can sometimes block blood vessels, these energy channels can also be blocked, and pranayama, among other practices, can help clear the passageways. As a whole, the nadi system makes sure consciousness and prana are carried to every cell. Of these thousands of nadis, we need to concern ourselves only with the three main nadis:

1. **Ida Nadi** – Terminating at the left nostril, *ida nadi* governs feminine energy and is cooling and receptive. It is also the activating channel of the right hemisphere of the brain.

2. **Pingala Nadi** – Terminating at the right nostril, *pingala nadi* governs masculine energy and is heating and active in nature. This nadi is the activating channel of the left hemisphere of the brain.

3. **Sushumna Nadi** – When prana is flowing evenly through the first two nadis, it can then enter the central channel, *sushumna*. This nadi is located along the center of the spinal column and is the channel through which consciousness can arise through the chakras.

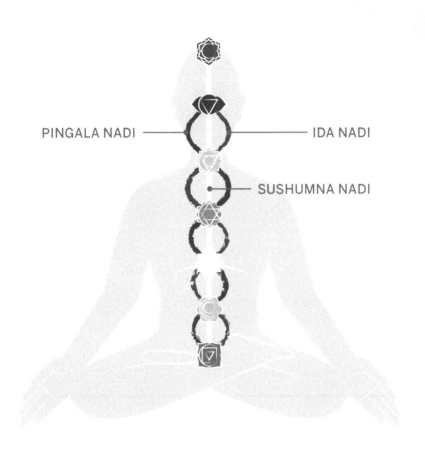

PINGALA NADI ——————— IDA NADI

——— SUSHUMNA NADI

The Chakras

Chakras are tiny spinning vortices throughout the body containing prana and aspects of mind. Though there are many chakras, we'll concern ourselves with only the seven main chakras, which run along the sushumna nadi. The first six are intersection points of all three nadis, while the seventh is the highest point of sushumna nadi. When the energy in all seven chakras is balanced and the nadis are clear, pure consciousness can move upward through sushumna, piercing each chakra and awakening higher consciousness.

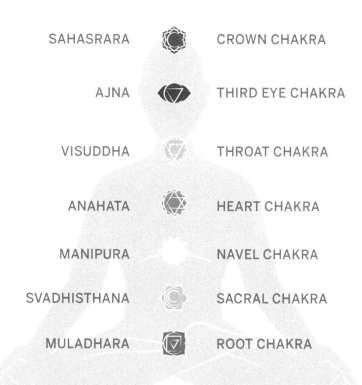

SAHASRARA		CROWN CHAKRA
AJNA		THIRD EYE CHAKRA
VISUDDHA		THROAT CHAKRA
ANAHATA		HEART CHAKRA
MANIPURA		NAVEL CHAKRA
SVADHISTHANA		SACRAL CHAKRA
MULADHARA		ROOT CHAKRA

Pranayama can intentionally move prana to chakras, stimulating them into a more balanced state. In this psychology, aspects of your mind are also stored in the chakras, so creating balance in the chakras creates balance in your mind.

1. **Muladhara (Root)** – Located at the center of the perineum for men and the tip of the cervix for women, *Muladhara* is the foundation of all chakras, governing your need for basic stability, survival, tribalism, and overall safety. For the health of the system to operate functionally, this energy center has to be balanced.

2. **Svadhisthana (Sacral)** – Located at the base of your spine, *Svadhisthana* is the center of preference, governing attraction, repulsion, creativity, sensuality, sexuality, rejuvenation, and

delight in the senses. Your identity starts being defined in this center as you decide what you do and don't like.

3. **Manipura (Navel)** – Located at the navel, *Manipura* is the seat of fire and clarity, governing self-esteem, empowerment, confidence, commitment, and decisiveness. It is the radiant splendor of your personality and the center for transformation.

4. **Anahata (Heart)** – Located at the center of your chest, *Anahata* is your spiritual center where no pain can enter, governing compassion, acceptance, forgiveness, joy, peace, and wisdom.

5. **Visuddha (Throat)** – Located at the center of the throat, *Visuddha* is the seat of truth, governing communication, reason, self-expression, and truth. It is the balancing point between the heart and the head and is a purified expression of the second chakra.

6. **Ajna (Third Eye)** – Located at the center of the brain, *Ajna* is the seat of intuition and higher knowledge, governing cognition, visualization, imagination, perception, clairvoyance, and intuition.

7. **Sahasrara (Crown)** – Located at the top of your head, *Sahasrara* is the point of transcendence, governing connection to divinity, cosmic consciousness, the transcendence of space and time, and boundlessness. Sahasrara opens only when all the chakras are in balance.

There are more than just these main seven chakras. Another chakra often mentioned is the *Bindu visarga*, located at the highest point on the back of your head. When the Bindu visarga is balanced and open, divine inspiration is able to flow down freely into our human consciousness.

The Bandhas

The *bandhas* are energy locks, or ways of collecting energy in the body. Since prana is continuously flowing, the three energy locks help capture it in certain regions of the system to concentrate prana. This will help direct it through specific nadis to specific chakras, or to change or direct the vayu.

1. **Jalandhara Bandha** – The chin lock, capping energy at the throat. With a tall spine, the head is pulled back slightly, the back of the neck is stretched, and then the chin is lowered. *Jalandhara Bandha* is engaged on the inhalation. It's important to note all steps and to not just drop the chin down.

2. **Uddiyana Bandha** – The navel lock, trapping energy at the mid-region of the body. With an exhalation, contract the abdomen toward the spine, feel your diaphragm rise and your lower abdominal muscles pull upward and inward, creating a hollow abdomen. For the beginner, *Uddiyana Bandha* can be engaged only with the exhalation.

3. **Mula Bandha** – The root lock, capping energy at the base of the body. This bandha is a subtle and upward contraction of the perineum toward the navel center. *Mula Bandha* is easiest to engage on the exhalation but can be maintained for the entirety of the breath.

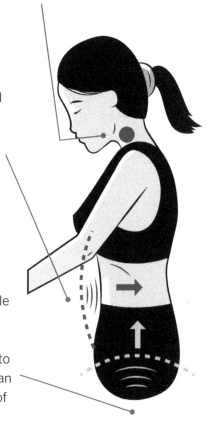

HOW IT WORKS

There are two primary ways to think about pranayama and its effect on the body, the energy, and the mind: the yogic perspective and the modern scientific perspective. While the ancients knew about these techniques and their effects long ago, studies in modern science are only now finding corroborative proof of pranayama's overall benefits.

The Yogic Perspective

Through the directional channeling of prana, pranayama can boost your immune system, clear your mind, help heal your body, and give you access to the wisdom within you. When you find yourself feeling sluggish and lethargic, you can turn to techniques that will help energize you. When you're feeling frenetic and restless, there are techniques you can use to calm the body, energy, and mind. The main goal from this perspective is to create harmony and balance throughout your entire system.

As with many yogic wellness practices, pranayama can often be used as preventive care. For example, if you are affected by seasonal affective disorder every winter, you can practice certain techniques that will help energize you and create heat in your system. When responding to symptoms of illness or allergies, you can use pranayama techniques to help cleanse the body of toxins.

The Modern Scientific Perspective

In recent years, scientists have come to understand that consciously controlling your breath can have huge benefits on your overall system, primarily with regard to the regulation of your nervous system in relation to anxiety, depression, and restlessness.

The vagal response is the stimulation of the vagus nerve, which runs down along the anterior portion of your spine from your brain to your internal organs. When the vagus nerve is stimulated, a signal is sent to the brain to reduce your blood pressure and calm your body and mind, reducing stress and helping to manage chronic illness, as healing can happen only in a more relaxed state of being.

For example, if your amygdala, the nerve center at the lower-central part of your brain, is agitated, it triggers your sympathetic nervous system (SNS) and your fight-or-flight response. You may become anxious, fearful, reactive, or frozen. Once triggered, this response lasts at least 20 minutes, but you can often find yourself stuck in this state for much longer. According to Dr. Mladen Golubic, an internist at Cleveland Clinic's Center for Integrative Medicine, when in this state, you take shallow chest breaths, sometimes halting the breath completely, extending the effects of your SNS response. By taking deeper and fuller breaths, especially by allowing the abdomen to relax and expand, the vagus nerve is stimulated, and calm can quickly be restored.

This calming and stress-reducing response is called the parasympathetic nervous system (PNS) response, or vagal response. When your SNS is calmed, you have more access to the prefrontal cortex of your brain, boosting your ability to think clearly and rationalize. Dr. Golubic goes on to say, "The vagal response reduces stress. It reduces our heart rate and blood pressure." This regulation of the nervous system is one of the primary benefits of a consistent pranayama practice.

THE BENEFITS OF PRANAYAMA

The benefits of a consistent pranayama practice are vast, including increased physical, emotional, mental, and spiritual well-being. Whether you are seeking to clear your mind, relax your body and mind, strengthen your breath and body, or connect with something higher than yourself, pranayama has a practice for you. Let's take a look at some of the benefits of a pranayama practice in detail.

Physical Benefits

Because of the physical components of pranayama, there are many benefits for your body, especially from an ongoing practice. Some techniques assist with efficient digestion: Regulating the breath directs the diaphragm, which pulses on the internal organs beneath it, which helps stimulate them into efficiency and massage away blocks in the digestive system. Some techniques clear your respiratory system, aiding with the elimination of toxins in the lungs, nasal cavities, and airways. Pranayama can even help with cardiovascular issues, as some techniques help slow down and regulate your heart rate.

When pranayama is combined with yoga postures, some benefits can be heightened. For example, taking full breaths in a posture can create more spinal extension, which can help reverse chronic misalignments (such as kyphosis and scoliosis).

Again, it's important to note that pranayama techniques are not cures or treatment plans for diseases. These techniques are meant to assist in your general care and can be used preventively.

Mental and Emotional Benefits

Because of pranayama's overall effect on the nervous system, there are many mental and emotional benefits to practicing. The first is that it can calm your mind. When your mind is running fast and it's hard to focus, these practices ground the mind in the present moment. This helps manage and reduce negative stress and anxiety as you pull yourself out of harmful or unhelpful psychological patterns. Also, because of this effect, pranayama techniques are essential to preparing the mind to go into deep states of meditation.

The more-stimulating pranayama practices can help with mental-emotional imbalances, such as chronic depression. By activating the nervous system in a systematic and balanced way, these techniques can clear the mental fog, redirect thoughts away from harmful ideas, and give you more energy to move past lethargy and sluggishness.

Spiritual Benefits

In the spiritual system of yoga, pranayama is one of the eight limbs on the yogic path to consciousness. By controlling the energetic flow in your body, you can clear the nadis and create balance in the chakras to bring about spiritual awakening. As you practice, you may begin to experience more spaciousness in your mind, allowing for clearer perspectives and connections to that which you hold divine.

Pranayama and Pain

You now know that breathing deeply can help you calm down, but did you know it actually changes the chemistry in your body? If you're not breathing enough or are breathing too shallowly because of anxiety, stress, or just bad breathing habits, not enough of the oxygen you inhale is converted to carbon dioxide, and the pH of your blood rises from 7.4 to 7.5 or 7.6. This is called hypocapnia, and it has a vasoconstrictive effect, meaning it narrows your blood vessels and restricts normal blood flow. You may have noticed a more extreme version of its effects if you've ever held your breath for an extended period or hyper-ventilated during a panicky moment: lightheadedness, dizziness, heart palpitations, and cold hands and feet. But since hypocapnia affects all your blood vessels, it's doing the same thing to every part of your body. That means your muscles are having their own version of lightheadedness or heart palpitations: spasms, weakness, twitching, and, of course, pain. Most of us aren't walking around consciously holding our breath, but many of us are experiencing a sub-tler form of hypocapnia nearly all the time. So, pranayama or breathing exercises aren't just a good way to relax; they literally get your blood flowing and help both treat and prevent pain.

There are great benefits to learning pranayama from a teacher, including being able to ask them questions. However, many practices are achievable without a live teacher. The techniques shared in the beginner section of this book will guide you into a deeper understanding of pranayama, and with practice, you'll have the competency to progress to more advanced practices on your own.

WHAT YOU'LL NEED

In this section, we'll discuss the things you need in order to have an effective and comfortable experience with pranayama. Some of these offerings will be necessary, and some will be nice to consider as you progress along your pranayama journey.

Space

The technique you are practicing will determine the best space in which to practice. For deeper, more contemplative practices with lots of steps, it is best to practice in a space free of sensory distractions. A quiet room in your home or office would be an ideal location in this case.

Sometimes, especially when a quieter space is unavailable, you can definitely practice on the go—in your car or at your desk. Because of the calming effects of many techniques, you may want to practice them when you feel your stress or anxiety levels rise. In this case, stop wherever you are and breathe.

Time

The techniques offered in this book will give you an understanding of how much time you will need for practice. Generally speaking, the beginner practices are shorter, and the more advanced practices are longer. Also, as we'll discuss in chapter 6 (page 139), you can sequence techniques to make them shorter or longer.

Consistency is key for an effective pranayama practice. It is recommended that you practice every day at the same time, if you can manage it. Be realistic in your goals. If you find that you're having a hard time fitting pranayama into your day, then start with a smaller and shorter practice, regardless of your skill level.

Clothes

There are no specific clothes you need to practice pranayama. Just keep in mind that you want to be comfortable and the clothing should not be restricting, so your body can move freely. For example, if you're practicing diaphragmatic breathing, it would be restrictive to wear a belt. If you're practicing pranayama with yoga postures, you'll need comfortable and stretchy clothing.

Props

Depending on what posture you'll be practicing in, you may need any of the following props:

- Yoga mat
- Yoga blocks
- Blanket
- Meditation cushion
- Chair
- Yoga bolster

Not everything on the list will be necessary for you. As techniques are described throughout this book, I'll inform you of the best posture(s) for each practice, and you can decide which, if any, of these props will best support you.

Other Equipment

You may need some additional tools to help you on your pranayama journey. For timed practices, you'll need a timer. A great addition to your practice is to spend a few moments each day reflecting in a journal, noting your experience. Additionally, if you are practicing in a space with noisy distractions, having soft music playing in the background might be useful.

TIPS AND TRICKS

Often, there are small adjustments that you can make in your practice to make these techniques either more accessible or more comfortable for you.

Go at your own pace. I'll be giving specific instructions for the practices in this book, including how fast or slow you should breathe. If you're having a hard time reaching these goals, go at your own pace, maintain a balanced nervous system, and allow yourself to progress naturally. Slower is faster, as we say.

Should I eat beforehand? A good rule is to always practice pranayama on a low to empty stomach. Some techniques are completely safe regardless, like Natural Breathing (page 44), but others require space in your abdomen in order to practice efficiently and with comfort.

Extra Precautions

Just as not all medications are right for every person, not every pranayama technique will be right for you (at least not always). Some reasons to stop practicing or to adjust your practice include the following:

* Respiratory Illness
* Respiratory Allergies
* Unregulated High Blood Pressure
* Heavy Menstrual Cycle
* Pregnancy

If you are suffering from respiratory illness (pneumonia, cold, asthma) or allergies, you may need to adjust your practice or not practice pranayama altogether until your healing process allows it. A common ailment I hear is that one nostril might be clogged while the other is more clear. For this, I advise imagining air moving through both nostrils, regardless of physical airflow. Sometimes this alone will unblock the clogged nostril.

Some of the more vigorous practices, especially around the abdomen, may not be good for those who are pregnant or who are experiencing a heavy menstrual cycle. In these instances, depending on your level of practice, you could reduce the intensity of the practice.

One last note here: If the technique you're practicing makes you feel unwell in any way, stop the practice. As toxins are released and internal organs are stimulated, sometimes the physical effects are sudden. Taking care of yourself is the most important factor here. Trust your body.

Try a different position. I'll be giving you specific postures to practice these techniques in, but much of the time, you can adjust your pose to better suit you. If you have a hard time sitting comfortably on the floor, try sitting in a chair. Some techniques can be done sitting or lying down. I'll let you know when there's a variance.

BUILDING A PRANAYAMA PRACTICE

As I've mentioned, consistency in practice is where you'll see the lasting effects of pranayama. I recommend spending at least a few minutes each day practicing. The ideal time to practice is first thing in the morning, as the mind is less occupied and the stomach is emptier, but if that's not realistic, any other time during the day will work. The calming practices, for example, are great to do before bed.

As you adjust the flows of prana in your system, you're essentially rewiring your energetic makeup. Like training a puppy, having a set schedule and practicing regularly will ensure the changes take hold and stay. On average, it takes about 66 days, or two months, for a new habit to take hold. Keep at it, even when it gets tough or you become less interested.

Chapters 3 through 5 of this book will give you 45 techniques to explore, ranging from beginner to advanced. In chapter 6, we'll discuss how to sequence pranayama techniques that will help you achieve specific energetic effects, and help you experience the full benefits of pranayama.

two

THE BUILDING BLOCKS OF BREATH

In this chapter, we'll cover the building blocks of pranayama to equip you with the precise tools you need to practice these techniques with confidence. There are many aspects to breathing and many ways to breathe, as you will read. We'll also go over the proper way to support yourself while practicing, whether that's seated in a chair, on the ground, or in another posture. In the end, we'll discuss *mudras,* or hand gestures, that can energetically enhance your pranayama practice.

THE FOUR ASPECTS OF PRANAYAMA

Breathing may seem simple and lacking in complexity, but as you practice pranayama techniques, you will realize just how dynamic it can be. In understanding the significance of each of the four aspects of pranayama, you'll be better able to track your progress.

* **Pooraka (Inhalation)** – Drawing air and prana into the body via the breath. By lengthening the inhalation, you can increase the brahmana (energizing) effect, stabilizing low-energy imbalances (sluggishness, depression, apathy).

* **Rechaka (Exhalation)** – Expelling air and toxins from the body via the breath. The exhalation stimulates a langhana (calming) effect and is tied directly to your parasympathetic nervous system. By lengthening it, you stabilize frenetic and restless energetic imbalances (anxiety, overstimulation, manic stress).

* **Antaranga Kumbhaka (Retention after Inhalation)** – When you hold your breath after the inhalation, you stimulate the brahmana (energizing) effect. With practice, you'll be able to hold it for longer periods, but remember to honor the limits of your body in a given practice.

* **Bahiranga Kumbhaka (Suspension after Exhalation)** – When you hold your breath after the exhalation, you stimulate the langhana (calming) effect. This aspect of the breath is said to be the hardest to master, as your body naturally craves more breath. With practice, you'll be able to practice this aspect without anxiety.

Practicing either *kumbhaka* (breath retention) is a goal of many pranayama techniques, and you should practice toward this goal slowly and systematically. This way, you will practice kumbhaka without triggering your stress response. If you hold the breath for too long or when you're not ready, you will make yourself anxious, countering the intended effect of the pranayama.

THE MANY WAYS TO BREATHE

Anatomically, breathing is the filling and emptying of the lungs, but which muscles engage, which organs move, and which nerves are stimulated during the breath will determine the specific effects on your practice. Some ways to breathe, especially when done unconsciously (not pranayama), can create health issues or trigger anxiety. Some ways are more energetically and mentally stabilizing. You can also breathe to different parts of your lungs to trigger certain effects, as we'll discuss.

Diaphragmatic Breathing

Sometimes called belly breathing, the diaphragmatic breath is the softening of the muscles around your abdomen, allowing the breath to relax that region of the body. This way of breathing can be done in a formal pranayama practice, or it can be a spontaneous way of breathing when the mind and body are relaxed.

No matter where you are, you can practice breathing in this way. First, be aware of the region of your body between your rib cage and your pelvis. Often, we constrict and hold tight muscles in this area of the body. Allow them to relax so that the belly can expand forward on the inhalation without resistance. The exhalation is a simple relaxation of the breath, with a slight contraction of the navel toward your spine. Aside from consciously relaxing the abdomen, there is no effort in this breathing style.

We will discuss a more detailed way of practicing diaphragmatic breathing in chapter 3 (page 48).

With practice and as your nervous system becomes more regulated, you may find yourself naturally breathing in this way. Some benefits to diaphragmatic breathing include reduced stress and anxiety, a more focused mind, relief from insomnia, slower heart rate, and improved digestion.

Thoracic Breathing

When the diaphragm doesn't descend toward the abdomen as you inhale, the breath then expands into the rib cage and chest to compensate. There are both pros and cons to breathing in this way. When done intentionally and with a pranayama technique, this way of breathing can increase vitality and be stimulating to the nervous system. When done unconsciously, your breathing capacity drops, and shallow breathing can have negative long-term effects on your health, especially with regard to cardiovascular diseases like sleep apnea. This is why you don't want this way of breathing to be your default breathing pattern.

To practice thoracic breathing, become aware of your diaphragm. As you inhale deeply, instead of drawing the diaphragm downward, hold it steady and allow the filling of the lungs to expand into the ribs, feeling your rib cage expand forward and laterally. With your exhalation, allow the diaphragm to relax and the rib cage to contract. We'll discuss ways to employ thoracic breathing in specific pranayama techniques in chapters 3, 4, and 5.

Clavicular Breathing

When you inhale and neither the belly nor rib cage expands, the movement of the breath rises toward your collarbones (clavicles), creating the shallowest way of breathing. Though it is part of a full and deep breath, you don't want to rely on clavicular breathing as the only part of your breathing. As I mentioned with thoracic breathing, when we breathe in a consistent and shallow manner unconsciously, we put stress on the body, especially the heart and brain. Less oxygen is absorbed, and we become tired and mentally sluggish. We'll discuss specific pranayama techniques in chapters 3, 4, and 5, when it is appropriate to employ this way of breathing.

Paradoxical Breathing

Paradoxical breathing is another breathing rhythm that happens unconsciously and can have negative long-term effects on your overall well-being. A strange phenomenon occurs when you inhale, where the diaphragm draws upward, and instead of expanding as you inhale, the chest contracts. The reasons for this include trauma or injury to the chest wall, disruption of nerves in the diaphragm, and weak respiratory muscles. Signs that you may be breathing unconsciously in this manner include shortness of breath, hypersomnia, exhaustion, poor sleep quality, abnormally quick breathing, and reduced physical performance.

The good news is that consistent pranayama practice could help correct this unhealthy breathing pattern and may even reduce the negative effects it has caused already. As always, consult with your physician if you notice any long-term negative effects of paradoxical breathing.

"Breath is the bridge which connects life to consciousness, which unites your body to your thoughts."

—Thich Nhat Hanh

POSTURE

When practicing pranayama, the position of your body matters because it allows the effect of the practice to be pronounced. Most practices are done seated, while some are done in yoga postures or even in conjunction with movements. I'll inform you of the best posture for each technique throughout this book.

Sitting in a Chair

It may be a relief that you don't have to sit on the ground in order to practice pranayama efficiently. The mechanics of it come down to the tilt of your pelvis and the alignment of your spine. Pick a chair that has a flat seat (cushioned is fine), doesn't tilt on its own, and has a straight back.

1. Make sure both feet are placed flat on the ground (or on yoga blocks if your legs are shorter) with your knees stacking directly over the ankles.

2. Your knees should be on the same horizontal plane as the center of your pelvis in order to avoid cutting off circulation at the back of the legs.

3. Allow your pelvis to tilt forward slightly and feel your lower back and front abdominal muscles engaging. Be careful not to over-tilt the pelvis forward, creating an excessive curvature of your lower back. The lower back should feel engaged but not aggressively so.

4. Let the top of the spine or center of your brain float directly over the center of your pelvis without any rounding of the shoulders.

5. Relax your shoulders away from your ears, with your hands resting gently on your thighs or knees.

6. Lastly, feel the top of your head lift toward the ceiling and your chin draw backward toward your throat slightly.

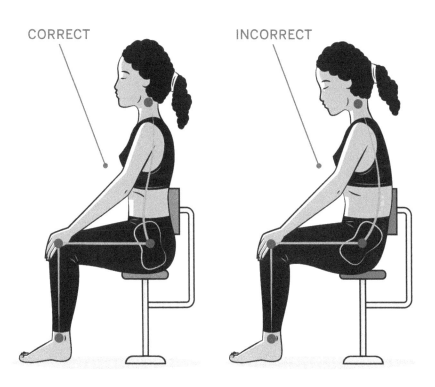

CORRECT

INCORRECT

Seated on the Floor

While there are advanced postures like Lotus pose to use when practicing pranayama on the floor, I'll describe here the most accessible seated postures for an effective pranayama practice. Our goal with posture is to make sure we can maintain the pose comfortably.

SIDDHASANA (ACCOMPLISHED POSE)

1. Come to sit on the floor with one leg crossed lightly over the other, with your top foot tucking toward your body.

2. Allow your spine to be tall, your pelvis to draw forward, and the top of your spine to float directly over the center of your pelvis. If you find difficulty drawing your pelvis forward (excessive rounding of your lower back), elevate your seat onto a meditation cushion, yoga block, or folded blanket.

3. Relax your shoulders down your back and allow your hands to rest on your thighs or knees.

SUKHASANA (EASY POSE)

1. Commonly referred to as sitting cross-legged, this pose entails sitting on the floor with your ankles crossed.

2. Follow the spinal alignment for *Siddhasana*, above.

3. Relax your shoulders down your back and allow your hands to rest on your thighs or knees.

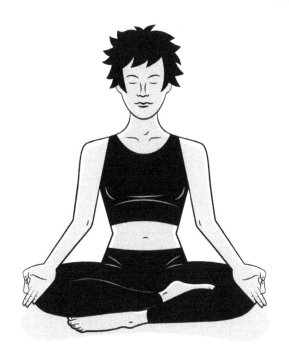

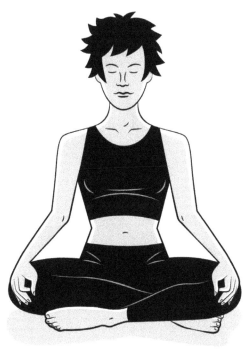

VIRASANA (HERO'S POSE)

1. Kneeling on the ground, sit so your feet come wide of your hips.

2. Follow the spinal alignment for Siddhasana (page 34). If you have discomfort in your knees or ankles, sit on a yoga block or cushion between your feet.

3. Relax your shoulders down your back and allow your hands to rest on your thighs or knees.

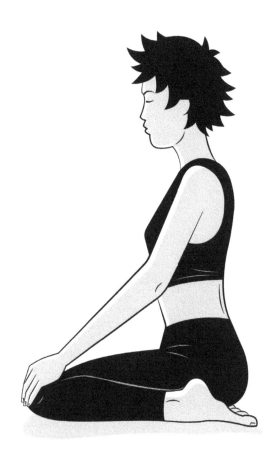

Lying on the Floor

Some pranayama practices can be done lying down (but ideally not in a bed, as our bodies associate beds with sleeping and you are more likely to fall asleep). *Savasana* (Corpse pose) is great for calming practices.

1. Lie down with your back and legs on the floor on top of a yoga mat or blanket.

2. Allow your arms to relax by your sides, palms facing upward, and your feet 12 to 24 inches apart, toes falling outward. If you experience discomfort in your lower back when lying down, tuck a yoga bolster beneath your knees to relieve pressure.

3. You may use a pillow or folded blanket beneath your head. Blocks and yoga bolsters are too high to use as pillows, as they put undue stress on your neck.

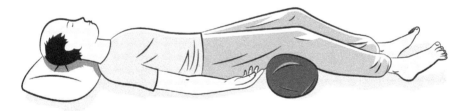

"The mind is the king of the senses, but the breath is the king of the mind."

— B. K. S. Iyengar

MUDRAS

The most familiar mudras are *hasta mudras*, or hand gestures, often used in meditation, pranayama, and asanas (postures). The word *mudra* in Sanskrit means "seal," and the gestures are used to enhance the effects of the flow of prana. Some gestures help calm your energy, some are uplifting, and some help connect you to something deeper than yourself.

There are many hand mudras, but four are more commonly used in pranayama, as I will describe here. As we move through the techniques, I'll suggest specific mudras to use to help enhance your practice.

Vishnu Mudra

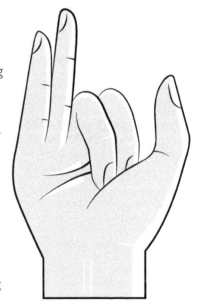

Vishnu Mudra is mostly used during the pranayama technique called *Nadi Shodhana*, which I'll describe variations of in chapters 3, 4, and 5. Regardless of your dominant hand, Vishnu Mudra is always practiced with your right hand, as it signifies the absorption of positive energy.

To practice Vishnu Mudra, raise your right hand and bend your index and middle fingers in toward your palm, leaving your thumb, ring finger, and pinky finger fully extended. This takes some dexterity, but it does get easier with practice.

Aside from its use in Nadi Shodhana to alternately block the nostrils, this mudra primarily balances the first three chakras (root, sacral, and navel centers). Because it is balancing to the base three energy centers, it also allows energetic access to the higher centers.

Gyan Mudra

Gyan Mudra is probably the best-known mudra, as it is used often in pictures and media representing yoga, Hindu, and Buddhist practices. It's also a fairly "safe" mudra to practice in any posture or practice. When in doubt, this is your go-to mudra.

With your palms turned upward on your knees, connect the tips of your pointer fingers to the tips of your thumbs on each hand. Allow the three remaining fingers to remain extended.

Gyan Mudra connects the tip of the pointer finger, which represents the lower mind or ego, with the tip of the thumb, which represents universal wisdom and consciousness. In essence, you are plugging into your higher mind and deeper knowledge. With the palms turned up on the knees, this is a more energizing mudra that opens you to receptivity.

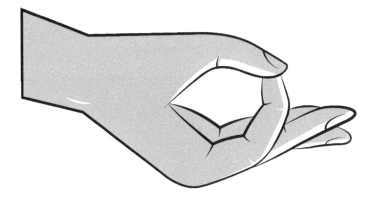

Chin Mudra

Chin Mudra, sometimes known as *Jnana Mudra*, is a simple hand gesture used for grounding during pranayama and meditation practices. Similar to Gyan Mudra, it is fairly universal and is a great complement to your practice.

Connect the pointer fingers of each hand with the tips of your thumbs, making a circle, leaving the three remaining fingers extended. Turn the palms downward on your knees.

Chin Mudra connects you powerfully to the root chakra, grounding you to the earth. When you're feeling frenetic, restless, and ungrounded, this mudra will help bring you back.

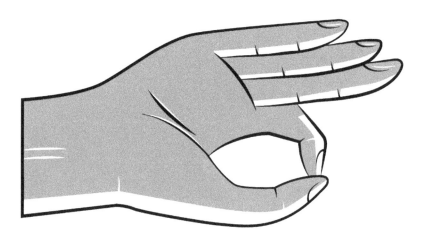

Anjali Mudra

Also referred to as prayer hands, *Anjali Mudra* can be used in pranayama and meditation, but it is also a common gesture of salutations or reverence in many cultures.

Sitting tall with your shoulders relaxed down your back, bring the palms and fingers together in front of your sternum or heart chakra, keeping the fingers pointing upward.

Anjali Mudra creates a balance between the body and mind, represented by the hands meeting at the center of your body. Along with connecting to your heart, this devotional mudra is all about connecting to a deep inner balance.

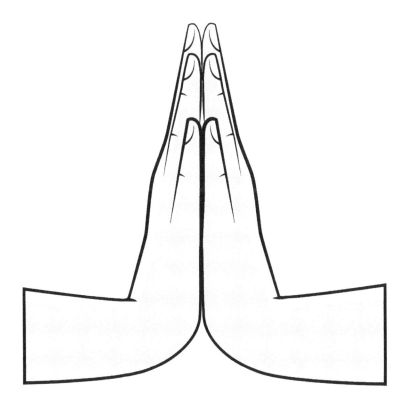

three
BEGINNER
(ADHAMA)

This chapter will cover foundational pranayama techniques that are vital to your practice. As you experience the effects of these practices, you'll return to them repeatedly, no matter how far your pranayama journey takes you. As you will see, some techniques offered later in this book are derivative of these basic techniques, so understanding them is absolutely essential.

These beginner-level practices are suitable for anyone wanting a window into the balancing, healing, and energetic effects of pranayama. Each one is meant to be practiced repeatedly, usually daily, until full mastery or comfort is established in the practice. Take your time, be patient with yourself, and, most important, just breathe.

NATURAL BREATHING
Journey of the Breath

TIME: 5 to 7 minutes
BENEFITS: Calming, Stress Relief

This foundational technique introduces you to your respiratory system and your natural breathing rhythm. Just this simple awareness, without any physical effort at all, will ground your mind and body. Given the low effort of this technique, it can be practiced virtually anywhere and in any posture.

1. In a comfortable posture, traditionally sitting tall or lying down in Savasana (page 37), allow your eyes to close, and relax your whole body.

2. Observe the instantaneous and natural rhythm of your breath, without trying to control the breath in any way, and feel it flowing through the nostrils on both your inhalation and exhalation. You may notice that the breath feels cooler during inhalation and warmer during exhalation. Continue for 10 effortless breaths.

3. Allow your awareness to trail to the back of your throat and notice the sensation of your breath as it moves in and out. Again, you may witness a difference in sensation between the inhalation and the exhalation. Continue for 10 effortless breaths.

4. Become aware of the region of your chest and rib cage. On the inhalation, notice the air moving through your trachea, into the bronchiole tubes, and feel the alveoli (air sacs) in your lungs inflate. Feel the lungs relax on exhalation. Continue for 10 effortless breaths.

5. Move your awareness to your abdomen. As the diaphragm pulls downward on the inhalation, feel the belly expand forward. As the diaphragm relaxes, feel the belly relax back toward the spine. Continue for 10 effortless breaths.

6. Finally, notice the entire relaxed breathing process in succession. As you inhale, first notice the breath in the nostrils, then the throat, then in the chest and rib cage, and then feel the abdomen expand. As you exhale, feel the abdomen relax, and the breath move out of the lungs, past the throat, and out of the nostrils. Continue for 10 to 20 more breaths.

   ☀ Simplified:
   • Inhale: Nostrils > Throat > Rib Cage > Abdomen
   • Exhale: Abdomen > Rib Cage > Throat > Nostrils

7. Feel your body as one single unit, breathing as one organ. Allow your eyes to gently open.

8. Journal your experience, noting any peculiar sensations, progress, and challenges.

   TIPS: Possibly the hardest part of this technique is staying present with the breath at each stage. Try counting the breaths backward from 10 in each step. If you're afraid you'll fall asleep during this practice (or any practice), set a timer to ease any time-management worries.

EXPANDED BREATHING
Fuller Breath

TIME: 5 minutes

BENEFITS: Energy, Mental Clarity, Improved Circulation, Increased Lung Capacity

This technique is energizing and helps stimulate the nervous system. Many people breathe just enough air to live. With practice, this technique will help you create a fuller natural breath capacity, giving more oxygen and nutrients to your entire system.

1. Set a timer for 5 minutes.

2. In a comfortable seated posture or lying on the floor in Savasana (page 37), allow your eyes to close, and feel your body relax.

    ＊ If you'd like, try using Gyan Mudra (page 39) or Anjali Mudra (page 41).

3. Bring your awareness to the movement of your chest and rib cage for five breaths, noting how deep or shallow your current breathing rhythm might be.

4. With a smooth and slow inhalation, allow your lungs to fill to capacity, almost to the point of straining.

5. Exhale slowly and completely.

6. Repeat steps 4 and 5 for 2 to 3 minutes.

   ※ As your lungs adjust to the new capacity, your breaths
   might become deeper every few rounds of breath. Keep the
   breath moving slowly.

7. Relax all effort and notice your breath adjust. Note how your
   breath may naturally remain at an increased capacity when
   the practice is completed.

8. Journal your experience, noting any peculiar sensations,
   progress, and challenges.

   TIP: Because of the effort to fill the lungs, sometimes
   your jaw will want to clench. Notice if that happens and
   consciously relax the jaw (or any other straining muscles).

DIAPHRAGMATIC BREATHING

Belly Breath

TIME: 10 minutes

BENEFITS: Calming, Stress Relief, Improved Digestion

Diaphragmatic Breathing stimulates the parasympathetic nervous system, drawing you out of stressful mind patterns and grounding you in the softness of your belly. If you find yourself agitated after a long day or unable to fall asleep, this technique is your go-to pranayama. This technique is also suggested as the best natural breathing rhythm to maintain a calm and steady mind.

1. Either in a seated posture or lying down in Savasana (page 37), close your eyes and feel your body completely relax.

2. Place your dominant hand lightly over your abdomen and feel your natural breath moving into your hand. Avoid pulling the belly in or pushing it out. Continue this awareness for five effortless breaths.

3. Soften any clenching, gripping, or holding in the muscles of your abdomen and pelvis. As those muscles continue to relax, without effort, the breath may naturally pool down into your belly. Continue to soften the belly for 2 minutes.

   ✳ At this point, you can release your hand to your knee (if seated) or to the floor (if lying down). If it is comfortable to keep your hand on your abdomen, then do so.

4. If it hasn't happened naturally already, relax the movement of your chest and rib cage, allowing the only movement of your body to the be the soft expansion and release of your belly.

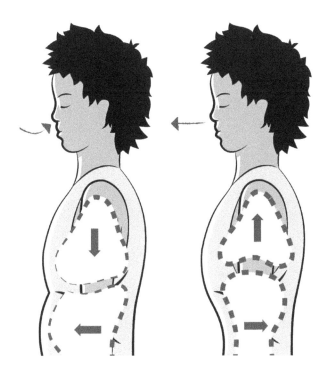

✳ If your mind wanders, the breath might creep back up into your chest. When that happens, relax all effort and see the breath return to the abdomen.

5. Try to keep the breath soft in your belly for 5 minutes.

6. When you feel complete in the practice, allow the eyes to gently open and stay present to the calming effect of the technique.

7. Journal your experience, noting any peculiar sensations, progress, and challenges.

TIP: Those new to this technique may find it difficult to relax the movement of the chest and rib cage, especially if they are in a stressed state. If this is the case for you, just do your best and continue to relax the abdomen. Eventually, it will relax.

MAKARASANA BREATHING

Calm Crocodile

TIME: 10 minutes
BENEFITS: Calming, Stress Relief, Restoration,
Improved Digestion

This technique amplifies the restorative effects of
Diaphragmatic Breathing (page 48) with the employment
of *Makarasana,* or Calm Crocodile pose. Breathing into
the belly while simultaneously resting on your abdomen
enhances the connection to your calming and grounded
nervous system. This technique is perfect if you're feeling
panicky, anxious, and restless.

1. Set a timer for 10 minutes.

2. Roll out a yoga mat and lie facedown on the floor with your
   arms crossed underneath your forehead. Have your elbows
   just a few inches forward of your shoulders so your chest rises
   from the ground slightly. Have your feet as wide as your yoga
   mat and allow the inside arches to rest on the ground, with
   your hips externally rotated and opening to the floor.

3. Allow your eyes to close, and relax your body, feeling your
   abdomen resting against the earth. Soften any clenching, gripping, or holding in the muscles of your abdomen and pelvis.

4. Without straining, notice your natural breath for 2 minutes.

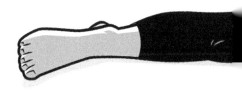

5. Begin to relax the movement of the breath down into your belly. Since the abdomen is resting against the earth, it may feel counterintuitive at first to breathe this way. It's okay to put some slight effort into bringing the breath there. Limit the movement of the chest and rib cage. Keep relaxing and keep the breath in your belly for 5 minutes.

6. Take a deeper, fuller breath and make small movements in your legs and feet as you bring yourself back. Rolling over onto your back, hug your knees into your chest for a few breaths to counterpose.

7. When you're ready, come to a seated position and notice the effects of the practice on your mind, energy, and body.

8. Journal your experience, noting any peculiar sensations, progress, and challenges.

TIPS: If it feels like too much effort or is uncomfortable to keep your elbows back and your chest lifted, roll a blanket up and slide it underneath your chest for support. If your forehead is uncomfortable on the backs of your hands or wrists, you can rest a blanket there as well.

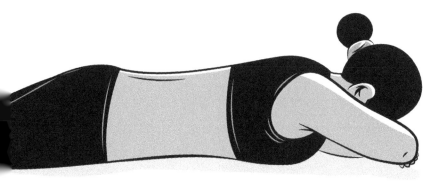

SAMA VRITTI
Balanced Breath

TIME: 5 minutes

BENEFITS: Calming, Balance, Mental Clarity, Improved Circulation

This standard technique balances the energy in your body and mind by evening out the length of the inhalation and exhalation. Sama Vritti is also the name of the energetic effect this technique offers (page 6), creating a calm and alert mind. When you're not sure which pranayama technique to practice, this one is always a safe bet.

1. Set a timer for 5 minutes.

2. In a comfortable seated posture or lying on the floor in Savasana (page 37), allow your eyes to close, and feel your body relax.

   ✳ If you'd like, try using Gyan Mudra (page 39) or Chin Mudra (page 40).

3. Notice the natural rhythm of your breath for 10 breaths, noting if your inhalation seems longer or shorter than your exhalation.

4. With a slow and steady inhalation, draw breath into your body for six counts of breath.

  ✳ A count of breath is an estimated 1 second, or the time it takes to chant "*Om.*"

5. Without pausing, slowly exhale for six counts.

6. Complete at least 12 rounds of this balanced breath.

7. Release the technique and feel your breath adjust. Allow your eyes to gently open.

8. Journal your experience, noting any peculiar sensations, progress, and challenges.

  TIPS: Though it takes some effort to even out the breath at first, you can relax that effort by slowing down the intake of breath on the inhalation and slowing down the output of breath on the exhalation. If you have a metronome, you can use that to help count the breaths.

RECLINED PURE BREATH
Ferris Wheel Breathing

TIME: 10 minutes

BENEFITS: Stress Relief, Restoration, Improved Digestion

The Pure Breath expands on both Diaphragmatic Breathing (page 48) and Sama Vritti (page 52). For this beginner version of the technique, you'll be lying on the floor in Savasana (page 37) to allow optimal relaxation of the body and breath, grounding your energy and harmonizing your mind.

1. Set a timer for 10 minutes.

2. Lie on the floor atop a yoga mat in Savasana, bringing a blanket under your head to make yourself more comfortable. Allow your arms and legs to relax open.

   ☀ Note: You can also practice this technique in Makarasana, or Calm Crocodile pose (page 50).

3. Bring your awareness to your breath, and begin to practice diaphragmatic breathing, softening the effort in your abdomen and pelvis to allow the breath to pool into the lowest portion of your lungs. Allow the belly to rise gently on the inhalation and relax toward your spine on the exhalation. Feel the chest and rib cage cease movement and relax into this technique for 2 minutes.

4. Keeping your breath grounded in your abdomen, now engage sama vritti by making sure the inhalation and exhalation are of equal length and quality. You can count the breath to help ensure its evenness. Breathe evenly to your belly for 2 minutes.

5. Continuing to breathe evenly to your abdomen, notice any hesitations, stoppages, or inconsistencies in your breath. Through relaxing the breath, start to iron out these "ripples" to create a smooth and even abdominal inhalation and a smooth and even abdominal exhalation. Continue this smooth, even abdominal breath for 2 minutes.

6. Again, keeping the previous breathing rhythms intact, become aware of the transitions between your breaths (the top of the inhalation and the bottom of the exhalation). At the top of your inhalation, relax all effort, allowing the inhalation to move seamlessly into the exhalation without really stopping. At the bottom of your exhalation, relax all effort, allowing the exhalation to seamlessly move into the inhalation without stopping. Continue this relaxed cyclical breathing for 3 minutes.

   ☀ To help envision the Pure Breath, think of a Ferris wheel continuously moving. On the inhalation, it rises to the top, and without stopping, it moves into the descent, the exhalation, and vice versa.

7. Take a deep breath and roll to your right side. After a few breaths, come to a seat and feel the energetic effects of the practice on your mind and body.

8. Journal your experience, noting any peculiar sensations, progress, and challenges.

   TIPS: If you feel you need more time in this practice, set your timer for longer. It's even more restorative to remain lying down for a few minutes after you've completed the technique.

DIRGHA PRANAYAMA
Three-Part Yogic Breathing

TIME: 10 minutes

BENEFITS: Energy, Improved Circulation, Increased Lung Capacity

Dirgha Pranayama combines diaphragmatic breathing (page 30), thoracic breathing (page 30), and clavicular breathing (page 31) in succession to create a full and controlled breath, systematically filling and emptying the lungs. If you're experiencing fatigue, poor posture, or depression, this technique will help uplift you.

1. Set a timer for 10 minutes.

2. In a comfortable seated posture or lying on the floor, allow your eyes to close, and feel your body relax.

   ✳ If you'd like, try using Gyan Mudra (page 39), Chin Mudra (page 40), or Anjali Mudra (page 41).

3. Become aware of the movement of your abdomen, feeling the belly fill and empty on the rhythm of your breath, holding this awareness for 1 minute.

4. Move your awareness to the widening and narrowing of your rib cage as you breathe, feeling the intercostal muscles between the ribs flex and release, for 1 minute.

5. Raise your awareness higher, feeling the slight lifting and lowering of your collarbones on the inhalation and exhalation. Because this section of the lungs is smaller, this movement will be the least pronounced. Hold this awareness for 1 minute.

6. With an exhalation, push all the air out of your body slowly.

7. As you inhale, first feel your abdomen expand, then your rib cage widen, and at the top of your inhalation, feel the collarbones lift. With your slow and controlled exhalation, feel your collarbones drop, then your rib cage narrow, and, lastly, feel your abdomen relax toward your spine. Continue this breathing rhythm for 5 minutes.

   ☀ Simplified:
   • Inhalation: Abdomen > Rib Cage > Collarbones
   • Exhalation: Collarbones > Rib Cage > Abdomen

8. Allow your breath to relax and notice the energetic effects on your mind and body. Allow your eyes to gently open.

9. Journal your experience, noting any peculiar sensations, progress, and challenges.

   TIP: If you're having a hard time compartmentalizing the breath in separate regions, you can imagine that the breath is moving up your spine as you inhale and moving down your spine as you exhale. With practice, sectioning out the breath will become easier.

CALMING UJJAYI PRANAYAMA

Ocean Breath

TIME: 10 minutes

BENEFITS: Calming, Improved Focus, Improved Circulation

This variation of *Ujjayi* calms the many movements of your mind to create better focus. By lightly making the breath audible, it draws the attention of your mind through sound, movement, and physical sensation. This breath also helps tune out distractions from the environment around you.

1. Set a timer for 10 minutes.

2. In a comfortable seated posture with your spine erect, close your eyes and relax your body.

   ※ Employ Chin Mudra (page 40) if you'd like to enhance the grounding effect.

3. Bring your awareness to the sensation of your breath at the back of your throat.

4. Constrict the glottis, or back of the throat, slightly to make a soft hissing or ocean-like sound as you inhale and exhale. It can often sound like a soft snore. Take long, slow, deep breaths in and out with the sound.

5. Keeping the breath audible, inhale for a count of four and exhale for a count of four for five rounds.

   ☀ A count of breath is an estimated 1 second, or the time it takes to chant "*Om.*"

6. Extend your exhalation to eight counts by slowing down the output of air, keeping your inhalation at four. Continue this breathing rhythm with the audible breathing for 5 minutes.

   ☀ Simplified: Inhale (4), Exhale (8)

7. Release the technique and notice the effect of the practice on your body and mind. Allow the eyes to gently open.

8. Journal your experience, noting any peculiar sensations, progress, and challenges.

   TIP: For beginners, the audible inhalation can sometimes feel straining on your vocal cords. If that's the case for you, make the breath audible on only your exhalation until you are more accustomed to the technique.

SIMHASANA PRANAYAMA
Lion's Breath

TIME: 3 to 5 minutes

BENEFITS: Stress Relief, Detoxification, Toning

The hardest part of practicing Lion's Breath is to not laugh at the funny face you have to make when doing it. This forced breath exercise helps clear your lungs of toxins and bring balance to your throat chakra. If you're having a hard time speaking your truth, add this practice to your routine.

1. In a comfortable seated posture with your spine erect, close your eyes and relax your body. Turn your palms up on your knees and splay your fingers wide with your arms stretched out.

2. Take a deep and quiet inhalation through your nose.

3. Simultaneously, perform the following as you exhale:

   ✳ Open your mouth and stretch your tongue out, curling it down toward your chin.

   ✳ Open your eyes wide and cross them to look at the tip of your nose, if you can.

   ✳ Constrict the glottis to make a loud "haaaa" sound.

   ✳ As the diaphragm draws upward, collapsing the chest, exhale all the breath from the body, wheezing slightly toward the end.

4. Repeat steps 2 and 3 up to five times.

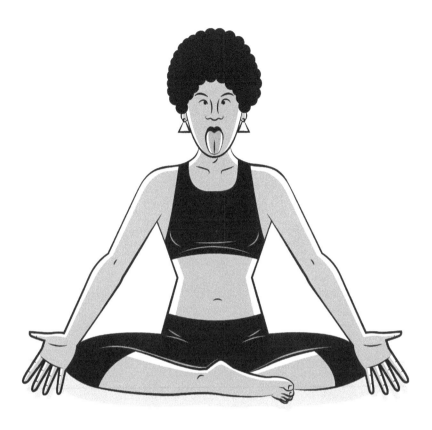

5. Rest for 1 minute with your eyes closed, paying attention to the movement of your chest and any sensations.

6. Journal your experience, noting any peculiar sensations, progress, and challenges.

   TIP: There are a lot of steps for the exhalation. Before you begin the technique, practice each of them individually to get a feel for them, which makes them feel more natural once you come into the practice.

BALANCING NADI SHODHANA
Alternate Nostril Breathing

TIME: 10 minutes
BENEFITS: Balance, Mental Clarity, Improved Focus,
Strengthened Intuition

Nadi Shodhana is a common pranayama that can be practiced in many ways, depending on your skill level and desired energetic effect. This variation brings your mind into sharp focus, balancing the activation of both hemispheres of your brain while stimulating the third eye chakra.

1. Set a timer for 10 minutes.

2. In a comfortable seated posture with your spine erect, close your eyes and relax your body.

3. Establish an even breathing rhythm (Sama Vritti, page 52), inhaling for a count of six and exhaling for a count of six. Continue for 2 minutes.

   ✳ Simplified: Inhale (6), Exhale (6)

   ✳ A count of breath is an estimated 1 second, or the time it takes to chant "Om."

4. Bring your right hand into Vishnu Mudra (page 38). When the practice begins, you'll alternate using your ring finger to block your left nostril and your thumb to block your right nostril.

5. Maintaining a six-count even breath, block your right nostril with your thumb and breathe in through your left nostril for six counts.

6. Release your thumb and block your left nostril with your ring finger. Exhale for six counts through your right nostril.

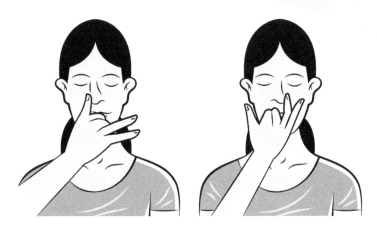

7. Keeping the right nostril open, inhale for six counts through the right nostril.

8. Block the right nostril, and open the left. Exhale for six counts through the left nostril.

   ✳ Simplified: Inhale Left (6), Exhale Right (6), Inhale Right (6), Exhale Left (6)

9. Repeat steps 5 through 8 for 5 minutes (for a minimum of six rounds).

10. Release the mudra and rest for 1 to 2 minutes with your eyes closed, aware of any sensations, especially at the center of your brain.

11. Journal your experience, noting any peculiar sensations, progress, and challenges.

TIPS: If one nostril is either partially or completely blocked, loosen the closed nostril slightly while still imagining air flowing through the opened nostril. Sometimes the right arm can get fatigued during this practice. To support it, allow the left arm to hug your body and rest your right elbow on top of the arm. If you have a cold or sinus infection, skip this technique.

CALMING NADI SHODHANA
Alternate Nostril Breathing

TIME: 10 minutes
BENEFITS: Calming, Stress Relief, Improved Focus

This variation of Nadi Shodhana focuses on the langhana (page 6), or grounding effect, of this technique by extending your exhalation. This is great to do before bed when experiencing insomnia, or when you really need to calm your mind.

1. Set a timer for 10 minutes.

2. In a comfortable seated posture with your spine erect, close your eyes and relax your body.

3. Establish an even breathing rhythm (Sama Vritti, page 52), inhaling for a count of four and exhaling for a count of four. Continue for 1 minute.

   ✳ Simplified: Inhale (4), Exhale (4)

   ✳ A count of breath is an estimated 1 second, or the time it takes to chant "*Om.*"

4. Extend your exhalation by slowing down the output of breath to a count of eight, keeping your inhalation at four. Continue for 1 minute.

   ✳ Simplified: Inhale (4), Exhale (8)

5. Bring your right hand into Vishnu Mudra (page 38). When the practice begins, you'll alternate using your ring finger to block your left nostril and your thumb to block your right nostril.

6. Maintaining the extended exhalation, block your right nostril with your thumb and breathe in through your left nostril for four counts.

7. Release your thumb and block your left nostril with your ring finger. Exhale for eight counts through your right nostril.

8. Keeping the right nostril open, inhale for four counts through the right nostril.

9. Block the right nostril, and open the left. Exhale for eight counts through the left nostril.

   ☀ Simplified: Inhale Left (4), Exhale Right (8), Inhale Right (4), Exhale Left (8)

10. Repeat steps 6 through 9 for 5 minutes (for a minimum of six rounds).

11. Release the mudra and rest for 1 to 2 minutes with your eyes closed, aware of sensation, especially at the center of your brain.

12. Journal your experience, noting any peculiar sensations, progress, and challenges.

TIPS: If one nostril is either partially or completely blocked, loosen the closed nostril slightly while still imagining air flowing through the opened nostril. Sometimes the right arm can get fatigued during this practice. To support it, allow the left arm to hug your body and rest your right elbow on top of the arm. If you have a cold or sinus infection, skip this technique.

KAPALABHATI

Shining Skull Breath

TIME: 7 to 10 minutes
BENEFITS: Energy, Mental Clarity, Detoxification

Kapalabhati helps cleanse the body of airborne toxins and clears the mind to make you alert and energized. You will feel less cloudy in your mind, creating a clearer perception of the truth around you. You might also feel a surge of energy that will carry you through your day.

1. In a comfortable seated posture with your spine erect, close your eyes and relax your body.

   ☀ If you'd like to enhance the energizing effect, employ Gyan Mudra (page 39).

2. Bring your awareness to your abdomen and feel your breath moving there for 1 minute.

3. Take a deep breath in through your nostrils, feel your abdomen expand, and then quickly and sharply exhale through both nostrils, feeling your navel pull back toward your spine. Inhale, allowing the inhalation to expand in the abdomen quickly but passively (like a balloon filling) and quickly exhale through both nostrils again, feeling the abdomen snap back.

   ☀ The physical engagement of this technique is similar to blowing out a candle, but with your mouth closed—actively exhaling and passively inhaling.

   ☀ Note that the movement of your body is isolated to the abdomen (see image). Breathing in your chest in this technique will lead to dizziness.

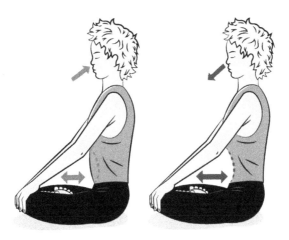

4. Repeat step 3 for 27 rapid breaths.

   ✳ If you experience dizziness, you may be breathing
   too forcefully. Slow down your pace and practice with
   less force.

5. After 27 breaths, relax the practice and feel your breath
   adjust, noticing sensations for a few moments.

6. Repeat steps 3 through 5 twice more (for a total of three
   rounds), taking a short break between rounds to notice
   sensations.

7. Sit quietly for 3 minutes and notice the sensations of the
   practice. You might sense light in your brain, warmth in your
   abdomen, and spaciousness in your lungs.

8. Journal your experience, noting any peculiar sensations,
   progress, and challenges.

   TIPS: Practice this technique at least 2 hours after eating. If
   you are pregnant, currently experiencing a heavy menstrual
   cycle, or have unregulated high blood pressure, you may
   want to skip this technique.

BHRAMARI PRANAYAMA

Buzzing Bee Breath

TIME: 5 minutes

BENEFITS: Calming, Stress Relief, Mental Clarity

Buzzing Bee Breath has a unique way of calming the body and mind by creating small vibrations in your brain and soothing your nerves. If you find that your mind just won't stop running, then this is the perfect practice for you.

1. Set a timer for 5 minutes.

2. In a comfortable seated posture with your spine erect, close your eyes and relax your body.

3. Place your index fingers onto the small triangular flaps in front of your ear canals (the tragi) and press them inward to block the ear canals. (Do not put your fingers directly into the ear canals.)

4. Inhale slowly and completely through both nostrils.

5. Exhale, pressing your tongue against the roof of your mouth, and start to hum loudly. Keep a continuous hum until you run out of breath.

   ✳ There are two ways to hum: making an "mmm" sound and making an "nnn" sound. For this technique, make a nasally "nnn" sound (as in the name Nancy) to hum. This will encourage the vibration at the center of your brain.

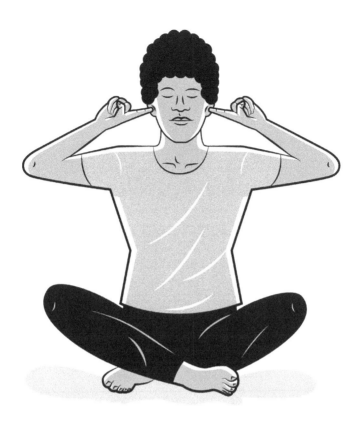

6. Repeat steps 4 and 5 for 2 to 3 minutes without pausing.

7. Stop humming and release your arms to rest on your knees. With the breath quiet, stay focused inward until you feel the desire to come back.

8. Journal your experience, noting any peculiar sensations, progress, and challenges.

   TIP: Because you'll be making sound, you may want to turn up the volume on your timer.

SHEETALI PRANAYAMA
Cooling Breath

TIME: 5 minutes
BENEFITS: Cooling, Calming, Improved Focus

Sheetali Pranayama reduces your body temperature and also calms fiery emotional states of mind such as anger and agitation. On a hot day, this is the pranayama you'll want to practice for staying cool, calm, and collected.

1. In a comfortable seated posture with your spine erect, close your eyes and relax your body.

    ☀ If you'd like to encourage the calming and grounding effect of this practice, employ Chin Mudra (page 40).

2. Stick your tongue out of your mouth and curl the sides up and inward to make a tube.

3. Inhale slowly through the tube, feeling the cool sensation on the tongue, saliva, and in the mouth and throat.

4. Close your mouth and press your tongue gently against the roof of your mouth as you quietly exhale through your nose.

    ☀ The silence of the exhalation is essential to maintain the cooling effect of this practice.

5. Repeat steps 3 and 4 for nine full rounds.

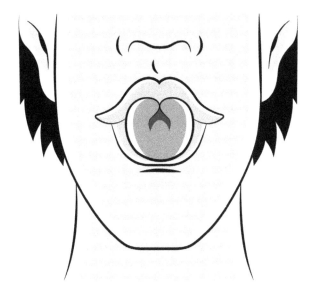

6. Rest and feel the cooling in your mouth, swallowing the cooler saliva, and allow the sensation to spread to your entire body.

7. Journal your experience, noting any peculiar sensations, progress, and challenges.

TIP: There are some people who are not able to roll the tongue into a tube. Don't be discouraged if that's the case. Simply move to the following practice, *Sheetkari Pranayama* (page 72), for similar benefits.

SHEETKARI PRANAYAMA
Hissing Breath

TIME: 5 minutes
BENEFITS: Cooling, Calming, Improved Focus

Sheetkari Pranayama is a cooling technique in which the mouth takes a special shape as you make the sound "shee" on inhalation, which is similar to a hiss. This is a great alternative to Sheetali Pranayama (page 70) if you're unable to roll the tongue into a tube. In addition to helping with cooling down during warm weather, this practice can also help reduce the symptoms of hot flashes.

1. In a comfortable seated posture with your spine erect, close your eyes and relax your body.

   ✳ If you'd like to encourage the calming and grounding effect of this practice, employ Chin Mudra (page 40).

2. Spreading your lips as much as you can comfortably, press the upper and lower rows of teeth together. Flip the tip of your tongue to the roof of the back portion of your mouth.

3. Inhale slowly through the teeth, making a "sheee" hissing sound.

4. Keeping the tip of your tongue flipped back, close your lips, and exhale quietly through your nostrils.

   ✳ The silence of the exhalation is essential to maintain the cooling effect of this practice.

5. Repeat steps 2 through 4 for nine full rounds.

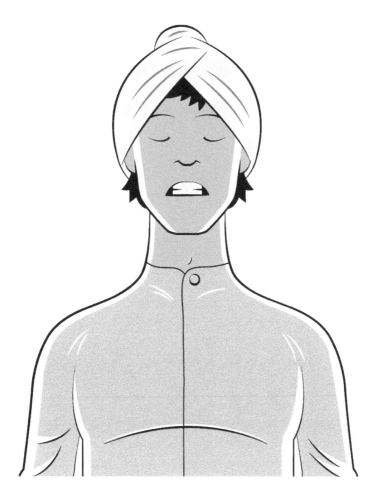

6. Rest and feel the cooling in your mouth, swallowing the cool saliva and allowing that sensation to spread to your entire body.

7. Journal your experience, noting any peculiar sensations, progress, and challenges.

   TIP: If your teeth are hypersensitive to cold, you may skip this technique or try the previous technique, Sheetali Pranayama.

four

INTERMEDIATE
(MADHYAMA)

In this chapter, you'll take your pranayama practice to the next level. After you've practiced the foundational techniques in chapter 3, you'll be able to advance to the intermediate techniques offered here. As you will see, many of these techniques are derivative or more advanced versions of their beginner counterparts.

Some new concepts that are offered in this chapter include breath retention, longer rounds of breathing, and combining breath with movement. As with the beginner techniques, the techniques offered here should be practiced repeatedly over time to achieve lasting benefits.

SEATED PURE BREATH
Ferris Wheel Breathing

TIME: 12 minutes
BENEFITS: Stress Relief, Improved Digestion

Blending Diaphragmatic Breathing (page 48) and Sama Vritti (page 52), this version of Pure Breath teaches you to remain calm and restful, even while physically engaged in a tall seat. As you sit, you'll need to isolate the muscles necessary for a supported seat while simultaneously softening the muscles of your front abdomen and the muscles of your pelvis.

1. Set a timer for 12 minutes.

2. In a comfortable seated posture with your spine erect, close your eyes and relax your body.

   ⁕ If you'd like to encourage the grounding effect, employ Chin Mudra (page 40).

3. Bring your awareness to your breath and begin to practice diaphragmatic breathing, softening the effort in your front abdomen and pelvis to allow the breath to pool into the lowest portion of your lungs. Allow the belly to expand gently on inhalation and contract toward your spine on exhalation. Feel the chest and rib cage cease movement and relax into this technique for 2 minutes.

4. Keeping your breath grounded in your abdomen, now engage sama vritti by making sure the inhalation and exhalation are of equal length and quality. You can count the breath to help ensure its evenness. Breathe evenly into your belly for 2 minutes.

5. Continue to breathe evenly to your abdomen, and notice any hesitations, stoppages, or inconsistencies in your breath. Through relaxing the breath, start to iron out these "ripples" to create a smooth and even abdominal inhalation and a smooth and even abdominal exhalation. Continue this smooth, even abdominal breath for 2 minutes.

6. Again, keeping the previous breathing rhythms intact, become aware of the transitions between your breaths (the top of the inhalation and the bottom of the exhalation). At the top of your inhalation, relax all effort and allow the inhalation to move seamlessly into the exhalation without really stopping. At the bottom of your exhalation, again relax all effort and allow the exhalation to seamlessly move into the inhalation without stopping. Continue this relaxed cyclical breathing for 5 minutes.

   ☀ To help envision the Pure Breath, think of a Ferris wheel continuously moving. On inhalation, it rises to the top, and without stopping it moves into the descent, the exhalation, and back up again.

7. Release the technique and feel your breath adjust. Allow your eyes to gently open.

8. Journal your experience, noting any peculiar sensations, progress, and challenges.

   TIP: It can be harder to maintain this practice while seated versus lying down. A good midpoint is to sit with your back against the wall. Keep the abdomen engaged but use the support of the wall to stay sitting tall.

BALANCING UJJAYI PRANAYAMA

Ocean Breath

TIME: 10 minutes
BENEFITS: Balance, Mental Clarity, Improved Focus, Improved Circulation

This balancing variation of Ujjayi adds kumbhaka, or breath retention (page 28). After establishing an even rhythm of breathing, you'll then insert short pauses between breaths as prescribed here. When you intentionally pause the breath, you begin to create the conditions necessary for the mind to become still.

1. Set a timer for 10 minutes.

2. In a comfortable seated posture with your spine erect, close your eyes and relax your body.

3. Bring your awareness to the sensation of your breath at the back of your throat.

4. Constrict the glottis, or back of the throat, slightly to make a soft hissing or ocean-like sound as you inhale and exhale. It can often sound like a soft snore. Take long, slow, deep breaths in and out with the sound.

5. Keeping the breath audible, inhale for a count of six and exhale for a count of six for five rounds.

   ☀ A count of breath is an estimated 1 second, or the time it takes to chant "*Om*."

6. Inhale audibly for a count of six.

7. Retain your breath in while engaging Jalandhara Bandha (page 14) by contracting your chin toward your throat for three counts.

8. Exhale audibly for a count of six.

9. Hold your breath out while pulling up Mula Bandha (page 14) by contracting the base of the body upward for three counts.

✳ Simplified: Inhale (6), Hold In (3), Exhale (6), Hold Out (3)

10. Repeat steps 6 through 9 for 5 minutes.

11. Release the technique and notice the effect of the practice on your body and mind. Allow the eyes to gently open.

12. Journal your experience, noting any peculiar sensations, progress, and challenges.

TIPS: Holding your breath is not a competition, and you shouldn't seek to do so for as long as you can in this technique. It might feel subtle, but stick to the prescribed rhythm. If holding the breath in or out makes you anxious or uncomfortable, omit the holds for today.

INTERMEDIATE CALMING UJJAYI PRANAYAMA

Ocean Breath

TIME: 10 minutes

BENEFITS: Calming, Improved Focus, Improved Circulation

This intermediate version of Calming Ujjayi Pranayama (page 58) adds kumbhaka, or holding of the breath (page 28), after exhalation. This method induces the langhana (page 6) or calming energetic effect, making this technique your go-to on stressful days, in the evening, or when you're having trouble sleeping.

1. Set a timer for 10 minutes.

2. In a comfortable seated posture with your spine erect, close your eyes and relax your body.

   ✳ If you'd like to enhance the grounding effect, employ Chin Mudra (page 40).

3. Bring your awareness to the sensation of your breath at the back of your throat.

4. Constrict the glottis, or back of the throat, slightly to make a soft hissing or ocean-like sound as you inhale and exhale. It can often sound like a soft snore. Take long, slow, deep breaths in and out with the sound.

5. Keeping the breath audible, inhale for a count of six and exhale for a count of six for five rounds.

   ✳ A count of breath is an estimated 1 second, or the time it takes to chant "*Om*."

6. Inhale audibly for a count of six.

7. Without holding the breath in, exhale audibly for a count of six.

8. Hold your breath out while pulling up Mula Bandha (page 14) by contracting the base of the body upward for three counts.

   ✳ Simplified: Inhale (6), Exhale (6), Hold Out (3)

9. Repeat steps 5 through 8 for 5 minutes.

10. Release the technique and notice the effect of the practice on your body and mind. Allow the eyes to gently open.

11. Journal your experience, noting any peculiar sensations, progress, and challenges.

TIP: Keep your breath audible the entire time. Sometimes when we're counting the breath, we lose parts of the practice. Stay engaged.

ENERGIZING UJJAYI PRANAYAMA

Ocean Breath

TIME: 10 minutes

BENEFITS: Energy, Mental Clarity, Improved Focus, Improved Circulation

This version of Ujjayi has a brahmana (page 6), or energizing effect, to it by introducing kumbhaka, or breath retention (page 28), after your inhalation. This is a great technique to practice in the morning or when you need a gentle energetic boost.

1. Set a timer for 10 minutes.

2. In a comfortable seated posture with your spine erect, close your eyes and relax your body.

   ☀ If you'd like to enhance the energizing effect, employ Gyan Mudra (page 39).

3. Bring your awareness to the sensation of your breath at the back of your throat.

4. Constrict the glottis, or back of the throat, slightly to make a soft hissing or ocean-like sound as you inhale and exhale. It can often sound like a soft snore. Take long, slow, deep breaths in and out with the sound.

5. Keeping the breath audible, inhale for a count of six and exhale for a count of six for five rounds.

   ✳ A count of breath is an estimated 1 second, or the time it takes to chant "*Om*."

6. Inhale audibly for a count of six.

7. Retain your breath in while engaging Jalandhara Bandha (page 14) by contracting your chin toward your throat for three counts.

8. Exhale audibly for a count of six, moving into the next inhalation immediately without holding the breath out.

   ✳ Simplified: Inhale (6), Hold In (3), Exhale (6)

9. Repeat steps 6 through 8 for 5 minutes.

10. Release the technique and notice the effect of the practice on your body and mind. Allow the eyes to gently open.

11. Journal your experience, noting any peculiar sensations, progress, and challenges.

TIPS: If you find it difficult to engage Jalandhara Bandha, practice the engagement to build muscle memory before you enter into this technique. If holding the breath in makes you uncomfortable, skip this practice for today.

INTERMEDIATE KAPALABHATI

Shining Skull Breath

TIME: 10 minutes

BENEFITS: Energy, Mental Clarity, Detoxification

This intermediate variation of Kapalabhati (page 66) extends the rounds of practice, toning your abdomen and cleansing your respiratory system of toxins. At the same time, this technique creates light in the brain and mind, providing access to clearer intuition and the perspectives of others.

1. In a comfortable seated posture with your spine erect, close your eyes and relax your body.

   ☀ If you'd like to enhance the energizing effect, employ Gyan Mudra (page 39) or Anjali Mudra (page 41).

2. Bring your awareness to your abdomen and feel your breath moving there for 1 minute.

3. Take a deep breath in through your nostrils, feel your abdomen expand, and then quickly and sharply exhale through both nostrils, feeling your navel pull back toward your spine. Allow the inhalation to expand in the abdomen quickly but passively (like a balloon filling) and quickly exhale through both nostrils again, feeling the abdomen snap back.

   ☀ The physical engagement of this technique is similar to blowing out a candle, but with your mouth closed—actively exhaling and passively inhaling through the nostrils.

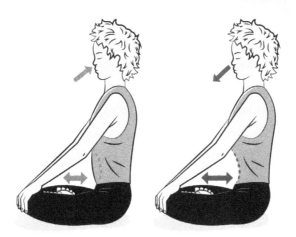

✳ Note that the movement of your body is isolated to the abdomen (see image). Breathing in your chest with this technique will lead to dizziness.

4. Repeat step 3 for 54 rapid breaths.

✳ If you experience dizziness, you may be breathing too forcefully. Slow down your pace and practice with less force.

5. After 54 breaths, relax the practice and feel your breath adjust, noticing any sensations for a few moments.

6. Repeat steps 3 and 4 twice more (for three total rounds), taking a short break between rounds to notice any sensations.

7. Sit quietly for 3 minutes and notice the sensations of the practice. You might sense light in your brain, warmth in your abdomen, and spaciousness in your lungs.

8. Journal your experience, noting any peculiar sensations, progress, and challenges.

TIPS: Practice this technique at least 2 hours after eating. If you are pregnant, currently experiencing a heavy menstrual cycle, or have unregulated high blood pressure, you may want to skip this technique.

CLARIFYING KAPALABHATI
Shining Skull Breath

TIME: 10 minutes
BENEFITS: Energy, Mental Clarity, Detoxification, Improved Focus

This variation of Kapalabhati (page 66) adds kumbhaka, or holding of the breath (page 28), after your final inhalation after each round. As you retain the breath, you are charging the clarifying and energizing effects of the practice. Practice this technique to help find the answers you seek when you find yourself in confusion and uncertainty.

1. In a comfortable seated posture with your spine erect, close your eyes and relax your body.

   ☀ If you'd like to enhance the energizing effect, employ Gyan Mudra (page 39).

2. Bring your awareness to your abdomen and feel your breath moving there for 1 minute.

3. Take a deep breath in through your nostrils, feel your abdomen expand, and then quickly and sharply exhale through both nostrils, feeling your navel pull back toward your spine. Allow the inhalation to expand in the abdomen quickly but passively (like a balloon filling), and quickly exhale through both nostrils again, feeling the abdomen snap back.

   ☀ The physical engagement of this technique is similar to blowing out a candle, but with your mouth closed—actively exhaling and passively inhaling through your nostrils.

＊ Note that the movement of your body is isolated to the abdomen. Breathing in your chest for this technique will lead to dizziness.

4. Repeat step 3 for 54 rapid breaths.

＊ If you experience dizziness, you may be breathing too forcefully. Slow down your pace and practice with less force.

5. After the final forced exhalation, inhale to fill your body, engage Jalandhara Bandha (page 14), and focus on light in your brain. Retain the breath until just beyond the point of comfort and then exhale slowly and with control.

6. Relax and feel your breath adjust, noticing sensations for a few moments.

7. Repeat steps 3 through 5 twice more (for three total rounds), taking a short break between rounds to notice any sensations.

8. Sit quietly for 3 minutes and notice the sensations of the practice. You might sense light in your brain, warmth in your abdomen, and spaciousness in your lungs.

9. Journal your experience, noting any peculiar sensations, progress, and challenges.

TIPS: Practice this technique at least 2 hours after eating. If you are pregnant, currently experiencing a heavy menstrual cycle, or have unregulated high blood pressure, you may want to skip this technique.

BHASTRIKA PRANAYAMA
Bellows Breath

TIME: 10 minutes

BENEFITS: Energy, Improved Digestion, Warmth

Bhastrika Pranayama is called the Bellows Breath because the belly is moving backward and forward forcefully like a bellows stoking a fire. In fact, that's exactly what you're doing during this practice, stoking your digestive and transformational fires while stimulating the navel chakra.

1. In a comfortable seated posture with your spine erect, close your eyes and relax your body.

    ☀ If you'd like to enhance the energizing effect, employ Gyan Mudra (page 39).

2. Bring your awareness to your abdomen and feel your breath moving there for 1 minute.

3. Take a deep breath in through your nostrils, feeling your belly fill and expand forward.

4. Exhale powerfully through your nostrils, feeling your belly empty and your navel contract back toward your spine.

5. Repeat steps 3 and 4 for 1 minute at a moderate pace.

    ☀ If you start to feel lightheaded, slow down your pace.

    ☀ Be mindful to keep the spine tall and as still as possible the entire time, especially in your lower back.

6. Relax and feel your breath adjust for a few moments.

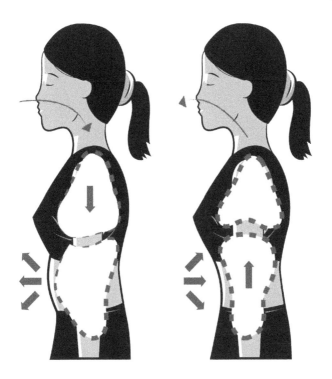

7. Repeat steps 3 through 5 twice more (for three total rounds), taking a short break between rounds to notice sensations.

8. Release the technique and sit tall, noticing any sensations for 3 minutes. Gently allow the eyes to open.

9. Journal your experience, noting any peculiar sensations, progress, and challenges.

TIPS: If you're new to this technique, go slowly at first to really get the mechanics of this practice down. As your competency grows, you'll be able to pick up the pace with more ease. Practice this technique at least 2 hours after eating. If you are pregnant, currently experiencing a heavy menstrual cycle, or have unregulated high blood pressure, you may want to skip this technique.

ROLLING BHASTRIKA PRANAYAMA

Fluid Bellows Breath

TIME: 10 minutes

BENEFITS: Energy, Improved Digestion, Warmth

Rolling Bhastrika Pranayama is a slow yet forced inhalation and exhalation from the abdomen. In this variation, you move your spine fluidly, like a snake, waking up the body and stimulating your chakras. If you're feeling stiff, especially in the cold of winter, give this technique a try.

1. In a comfortable seated posture with your spine erect, close your eyes and relax your body. Place your palms facing downward on your knees, lightly gripping them.

2. Bring your awareness to your abdomen and feel your breath moving there for 1 minute.

3. Take a deep breath in through your nostrils, feeling your belly fill.

4. Exhale powerfully through your nostrils, feeling your belly empty and your navel contract back toward your spine.

5. Repeat steps 3 and 4 for 10 rounds.

6. Next, with a powerful exhalation, rock backward slightly as you drop your chin, feel the chest contract backward, and feel the spine curve and the navel pull toward your spine until all the air is pushed out of your body.

7. Without holding the breath, inhale and rock forward, lifting your chin, feeling your chest expand and lift and your belly fill.

8. Repeat steps 6 and 7 for 20 rounds, continuing to move the spine forward and backward as you fill and empty the body.

   ✳ If you start to feel lightheaded, slow down the movement and breath.

9. Release the technique and sit tall, noticing any sensations for 2 to 3 minutes. Gently allow the eyes to open.

10. Journal your experience, noting any peculiar sensations, progress, and challenges.

TIPS: Anytime you combine your breath and your movement, it's a good idea to practice the movement apart from the breath to get the feeling into your body. Before settling into this practice, feel the spine snake forward and backward a few times. Practice this technique at least 2 hours after eating. If you are pregnant, currently experiencing a heavy menstrual cycle, or have unregulated high blood pressure, you may want to skip this technique.

INTERMEDIATE BALANCING NADI SHODHANA

Alternate Nostril Breathing

TIME: 12 minutes
BENEFITS: Balance, Mental Clarity, Improved Focus, Strengthened Intuition

This intermediate variation of Balancing Nadi Shodhana (page 62) adds kumbhaka, or breath retention (page 28), after both your inhalations and exhalations. Combined with Nadi Shodhana, the holding of breath helps still the mind, stoking your connection to intuition and clearer perception.

1. Set a timer for 12 minutes.

2. In a comfortable seated posture with your spine erect, close your eyes and relax your body.

3. Establish an even breathing rhythm (Sama Vritti, page 52), inhaling for a count of six and exhaling for a count of six. Continue for 2 minutes.

   ☀ Simplified: Inhale (6), Exhale (6)

4. Bring your right hand into Vishnu Mudra (page 38). When the practice begins, you'll alternate using your ring finger to block your left nostril and your thumb to block your right nostril.

5. Block your right nostril with your thumb and inhale through your left nostril for a count of six.

6. Close both nostrils and hold the breath in for a count of three while engaging Jalandhara Bandha (page 14).

7. Unblock your right nostril (leaving your left nostril blocked) and exhale for a count of six.

8. Close both nostrils and hold the breath out for a count of three.

9. Release the right nostril again and inhale through the right nostril for a count of six.

10. Close both nostrils and hold the breath in for a count of three, engaging Jalandhara Bandha.

11. Release your left nostril (leaving your right nostril blocked) and exhale for a count of six.

12. Close both nostrils and hold the breath out for a count of three.

   ✳ Simplified:
      • Inhale Left (6), Hold In (3), Exhale Right (6), Hold Out (3)
      • Inhale Right (6), Hold In (3), Exhale Left (6), Hold Out (3)

13. Repeat steps 5 through 12 for 8 minutes (for a minimum of six rounds).

14. Release the mudra, breathe through both nostrils, and rest for 1 to 2 minutes with your eyes closed, aware of any sensations, especially at the center of your brain.

15. Journal your experience, noting any peculiar sensations, progress, and challenges.

TIPS: If one nostril is either partially or completely blocked, loosen the closed nostril slightly while still imagining air flowing through the opened nostril. If you have a cold or sinus infection, skip this technique.

INTERMEDIATE CALMING NADI SHODHANA

Alternate Nostril Breathing

TIME: 10 minutes
BENEFITS: Calming, Mental Clarity, Improved Focus, Strengthened Intuition

With this version of Calming Nadi Shodhana (page 64), we add kumbhaka, or breath retention (page 28), after each exhalation to help induce the langhana, or calming energetic effect (page 6). If you find your mind racing, moving frenetically, or unable to stay focused, give this pranayama a try.

1. Set a timer for 10 minutes.

2. In a comfortable seated posture with your spine erect, close your eyes and relax your body.

3. Establish an even breathing rhythm (Sama Vritti, page 52), inhaling for a count of six and exhaling for a count of six. Continue for 2 minutes.

   ☀ Simplified: Inhale (6), Exhale (6)

4. Bring your right hand into Vishnu Mudra (page 38). When the practice begins, you'll alternate using your ring finger to block your left nostril and your thumb to block your right nostril.

5. Block your right nostril with your thumb and inhale through your left nostril for a count of six.

6. Release your right nostril while blocking your left and exhale for a count of six.

7. Close both nostrils and hold the breath out for a count of three.

8. Release the right nostril again and inhale through the right nostril for a count of six.

9. Release your left nostril and block your right and exhale for a count of six.

10. Close both nostrils and hold the breath out for a count of three.

    ☀ Simplified:
    • Inhale Left (6), Exhale Right (6), Hold Out (3)
    • Inhale Right (6), Exhale Left (6), Hold Out (3)

11. Repeat steps 5 through 10 for 6 minutes (for a minimum of six rounds).

12. Release the mudra, breathe through both nostrils, and rest for 1 to 2 minutes with your eyes closed, aware of sensations, especially at the center of your brain.

13. Journal your experience, noting any peculiar sensations, progress, and challenges.

TIPS: If one nostril is either partially or completely blocked, loosen the closed nostril slightly while still imagining air flowing through the opened nostril. Sometimes the right arm can get fatigued during this practice. To support it, allow the left arm to hug your body and rest your right elbow on top of the arm. If you have a cold or sinus infection, skip this technique.

ENERGETIC NADI SHODHANA

Alternate Nostril Breathing

TIME: 10 minutes

BENEFITS: Energy, Mental Clarity, Improved Focus, Strengthened Intuition

This energizing variation of Nadi Shodhana includes kumbhaka, or breath retention (page 28), after each inhalation, inducing the brahmana, or energetic effect (page 6). If you're seeking deep clarity, calm alertness, or illumination around a subject in your life, then this is the technique for you.

1. Set a timer for 10 minutes.

2. In a comfortable seated posture with your spine erect, close your eyes and relax your body.

3. Establish an even breathing rhythm (Sama Vritti, page 52), inhaling for a count of six and exhaling for a count of six. Continue for 2 minutes.

   ✳ Simplified: Inhale (6), Exhale (6)

4. Bring your right hand into Vishnu Mudra (page 38). When the practice begins, you'll alternate using your ring finger to block your left nostril and your thumb to block your right nostril.

5. Block your right nostril with your thumb and inhale through your left nostril for a count of six.

6. Close both nostrils and hold the breath in for a count of three while engaging Jalandhara Bandha (page 14).

7. Release your right nostril (keeping the left blocked) and exhale for a count of six.

8. Keeping the right nostril open, inhale for a count of six.

9. Close both nostrils and hold the breath in for a count of three, engaging Jalandhara Bandha.

10. Release your left nostril (keeping the right blocked) and exhale for a count of six.

   ✳ Simplified:
     • Inhale Left (6), Hold In (3), Exhale Right (6)
     • Inhale Right (6), Hold In (3), Exhale Left (6)

11. Repeat steps 5 through 10 for 6 minutes (for a minimum of six rounds).

12. Release the mudra, breathe through both nostrils, and rest for 1 to 2 minutes with your eyes closed, aware of any sensations, especially at the center of your brain.

13. Journal your experience, noting any peculiar sensations, progress, and challenges.

TIPS: If one nostril is either partially or completely blocked, loosen the closed nostril slightly while still imagining air flowing through the opened nostril. Sometimes the right arm can get fatigued during this practice. To support it, allow the left arm to hug your body and rest your right elbow on top of the arm. If you have a cold or sinus infection, skip this technique.

BALANCING KRAMA PRANAYAMA

Segmented Breathing

TIME: 10 minutes
BENEFITS: Calming, Balance, Improved Focus

Krama Pranayama takes kumbhaka, or breath retention (page 28), to a new level by inserting short pauses during your breath. These moments of stillness can halt the movement of prana and create the conditions necessary for a still mind. This balancing variation is a great go-to when your mind just won't turn off.

1. In a comfortable seated posture with your spine erect, close your eyes and relax your body.

   ☀ Employ Gyan Mudra (page 39) or Chin Mudra (page 40) if you'd like.

2. Bring your awareness to your natural breathing rhythm for 10 breaths, noting the current quality of your breath.

3. Begin a balanced breathing rhythm, inhaling for a count of six and exhaling for a count of six for 10 breaths. Noting the capacity of your breath, begin to identify where the halfway points are during your inhalations and exhalations.

4. Inhale to 50 percent of your breath capacity (three counts) and pause the breath for three counts. Inhale the remaining 50 percent of your breath (three counts) and pause with the breath held in for three counts.

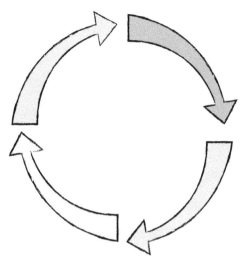

5. Exhale to 50 percent of your breath capacity (three counts) and pause the breath for three counts. Exhale the remaining 50 percent of your breath (three counts) and pause with the breath held out for three counts.

6. Repeat steps 4 and 5 for 10 breaths.

☀ Simplified:
- Inhale 50 percent (3), Pause (3), Inhale 50 percent (3), Pause (3)
- Exhale 50 percent (3), Pause (3), Exhale 50 percent (3), Pause (3)

7. Allow the breath to come to an effortless state and pay attention to any sensations, noticing a calmer and stiller mind.

8. Journal your experience, noting any peculiar sensations, progress, and challenges.

TIP: It can be easy to run out of breath or feel fatigued during this practice. If you find yourself straining at any point, take a break and return to the practice when your system has calmed.

CALMING KRAMA PRANAYAMA

Segmented Breathing

TIME: 10 minutes

BENEFITS: Calming, Improved Focus

This variation of Krama Pranayama (page 98) emphasizes the segmentation or pausing of the breath during your exhalation. This focus on the exhalation helps induce the langhana, or calming energetic effect (page 6). Especially if you find yourself ruminating on angry or anxious thoughts or emotions, give this intermediate technique a try.

1. In a comfortable seated posture with your spine erect, close your eyes and relax your body.

   ✳ Employ Chin Mudra (page 40) if you'd like.

2. Bring your awareness to your natural breathing rhythm for 10 breaths, noting the current quality of your breath.

3. Begin a balanced breathing rhythm, inhaling for a count of six and exhaling for a count of six for 10 breaths. Noting the capacity of your breath, begin to identify where the halfway points are during your inhalations and exhalations.

4. Inhale a full six-count breath with no retention.

5. Exhale to 50 percent of your breath capacity (three counts) and pause the breath for three counts. Exhale the remaining 50 percent of your breath (three counts) and pause with the breath held out for three counts.

6. Repeat steps 4 and 5 for 10 breaths.

☀ Simplified:
  • Inhale (6)
  • Exhale 50 percent (3), Pause (3), Exhale 50 percent (3), Pause (3)

7. Allow the breath to come to an effortless state and pay attention to any sensations, noticing a calmer and stiller mind.

8. Journal your experience, noting any peculiar sensations, progress, and challenges.

TIP: An added component to this practice is to imagine your thoughts dissolving during the pauses. Your mind may be moving immediately afterward, but you'll be training your thoughts to become still.

ENERGIZING KRAMA PRANAYAMA

Segmented Breathing

TIME: 10 minutes

BENEFITS: Improved Focus, Energy

As you focus on pausing the breath intermittently during the inhalation, this variation of Krama Pranayama (page 98) has a brahmana, or energizing effect (page 6). This is a great technique to practice when you're feeling sluggish, lethargic, or depressed.

1. In a comfortable seated posture with your spine erect, close your eyes and relax your body.

   ☀ If you'd like to enhance the energizing effect, employ Gyan Mudra (page 39).

2. Bring your awareness to your natural breathing rhythm for 10 breaths, noting the current quality of your breath.

3. Begin a balanced breathing rhythm, inhaling for a count of six and exhaling for a count of six for 10 breaths. Noting the capacity of your breath, begin to identify where the halfway points are during your inhalations and exhalations.

4. Inhale to 50 percent of your breath capacity (three counts) and pause the breath for three counts. Inhale the remaining 50 percent of your breath (three counts) and pause with the breath held in for three counts.

5. Exhale a complete six-count breath with no holds.

6. Repeat steps 4 and 5 for 10 breaths.

 ☀ Simplified:
  • Inhale 50 percent (3), Pause (3), Inhale 50 percent (3), Pause (3)
  • Exhale (6)

7. Allow the breath to come to an effortless state and pay attention to any sensations, noticing a calmer and stiller mind.

8. Journal your experience, noting any peculiar sensations, progress, and challenges.

TIP: Be careful not to hold the breath longer than prescribed, as doing so is not sustainable and can cause you to lose your breath over time. Even a short pause is effective during this technique.

SHEETALI ANULOMA PRANAYAMA

Cooling Alternate Nostril Breathing

TIME: 7 minutes

BENEFITS: Cooling, Stress Relief, Balance

This technique blends the cooling and calming effects of Sheetali Pranayama (page 70) with the balancing effects of Nadi Shodhana. This intermediate variation of these techniques is great for experiencing two practices working in tandem.

1. In a comfortable seated posture with your spine erect, close your eyes and relax your body. Bring your right hand into Vishnu Mudra (page 38) for the alternate nostril breathing portion of this practice.

2. Become aware of your natural breath for 10 rounds.

3. Stick your tongue out of your mouth and curl the sides up and inward to make a tube.

4. Inhale slowly through the tube, feeling the cool sensation on the tongue, saliva, mouth, and throat.

5. Unroll your tongue. Block your right nostril with your thumb and exhale slowly through your left nostril.

6. Roll your tongue again and inhale slowly through the tube.

7. Block your left nostril with your ring finger and exhale slowly through your right nostril.

8. Repeat steps 3 through 7 for 5 minutes.

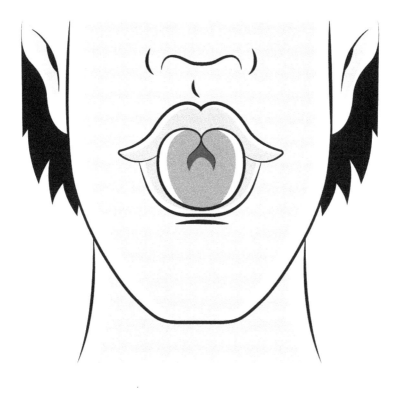

9. Release the technique and feel the cooling, calming, and balancing sensations in your body and mind.

10. Journal your experience, noting any peculiar sensations, progress, and challenges.

TIP: If you're unable to roll the tongue into a tube, you can do this same technique with the mouth in the position of Sheetkari Pranayama (page 72).

five
ADVANCED
(UTTAMA)

In this chapter, we'll cover advanced pranayama techniques. These practices help heal and balance your body, energy, and mind in profound and transformative ways, taking everything you've practiced in the last two chapters and building upon it. Some of the techniques are expanded or advanced versions of earlier practices, and some are brand new to this chapter.

On your pranayama journey, you'll spend a lot of time building toward these powerful techniques, mastering the practices of the beginner and intermediate chapters, and your work will be well worth the effort. Your energy body will shift as your nadis clear and your chakras balance, and you'll physically strengthen your respiratory system as well, allowing you stronger control for the techniques listed here, including kumbhaka, or breath retention (page 28).

ADVANCED BALANCING NADI SHODHANA

Alternate Nostril Breathing

TIME: 15 minutes

BENEFITS: Balance, Mental Clarity, Improved Focus, Strengthened Intuition

This advanced version of Balancing Nadi Shodhana (page 62) extends the breath even longer than earlier practices and continues the use of kumbhaka, or breath retention (page 28). The hyperfocus of the mind on counting breaths and controlling the flow of prana will stabilize negative mental patterns and give you stronger clarity.

1. Set a timer for 15 minutes.

2. In a comfortable seated posture with your spine erect, close your eyes and relax your body.

3. Establish an even breathing rhythm (Sama Vritti, page 52), inhaling for a count of six and exhaling for a count of six. Continue for 2 minutes.

   ✳ Simplified: Inhale (6), Exhale (6)

4. Extend your breathing to an eight-count even breath. Continue for 2 minutes.

   ✳ Simplified: Inhale (8), Exhale (8)

5. Bring your right hand into Vishnu Mudra (page 38). Block your right nostril with your thumb and inhale through your left nostril for a count of eight.

6. Close both nostrils and hold the breath in for a count of four while engaging Jalandhara Bandha (page 14).

7. Unblock your right nostril (leaving your left nostril blocked) and exhale for a count of eight.

8. Close both nostrils and hold the breath out for a count of four.

9. Release the right nostril again and inhale through the right nostril for a count of eight.

10. Close both nostrils and hold the breath in for a count of four, engaging Jalandhara Bandha.

11. Release your left nostril (leaving your right nostril blocked) and exhale for a count of eight.

12. Close both nostrils and hold the breath out for a count of four.

   ✳ Simplified:
     • Inhale Left (8), Hold In (4), Exhale Right (8), Hold Out (4)
     • Inhale Right (8), Hold In (4), Exhale Left (8), Hold Out (4)

13. Repeat steps 5 through 12 for 8 minutes (for a minimum of six rounds).

14. Release the mudra, breathe through both nostrils, and rest for 1 to 2 minutes with your eyes closed, being aware of any sensations, especially at the center of your brain.

15. Journal your experience.

   TIPS: If one nostril is either partially or completely blocked, loosen the closed nostril slightly while still imagining air flowing through the opened nostril. If you have a cold or sinus infection, skip this technique.

ADVANCED CALMING NADI SHODHANA

Alternate Nostril Breathing

TIME: 15 minutes
BENEFITS: Calming, Mental Clarity, Improved Focus, Strengthened Intuition

This advanced variation of Calming Nadi Shodhana (page 64) extends the breath, including kumbhaka, or breath retention (page 28), to further induce the langhana energetic effect (page 6). In the stillness between breaths, with prana halted, you can find expansive peace of mind.

1. Set a timer for 15 minutes.

2. In a comfortable seated posture with your spine erect, close your eyes and relax your body.

3. Establish an even breathing rhythm (Sama Vritti, page 52), inhaling for a count of six and exhaling for a count of six. Continue for 2 minutes.

   ✳ Simplified: Inhale (6), Exhale (6)

4. Extend your breathing to an eight-count even breath. Continue for 2 minutes.

   ✳ Simplified: Inhale (8), Exhale (8)

5. Bring your right hand into Vishnu Mudra (page 38). Block your right nostril with your thumb and inhale through your left nostril for a count of eight.

6. Release your right nostril while blocking your left and exhale for a count of eight.

7. Close both nostrils and hold the breath out for a count of eight.

8. Release the right nostril again and inhale through the right nostril for a count of eight.

9. Release your left nostril and block your right and exhale for a count of eight.

10. Close both nostrils and hold the breath out for a count of eight.

※ Simplified:
  • Inhale Left (8), Exhale Right (8), Hold Out (8)
  • Inhale Right (8), Exhale Left (8), Hold Out (8)

11. Repeat steps 5 through 10 for 6 minutes (for a minimum of six rounds).

12. Release the mudra, breathe through both nostrils, and rest for 1 to 2 minutes with your eyes closed, aware of any sensations, especially at the center of your brain.

13. Journal your experience, noting any peculiar sensations, progress, and challenges.

TIPS: If one nostril is either partially or completely blocked, loosen the closed nostril slightly while still imagining air flowing through the opened nostril. Sometimes the right arm can get fatigued during this practice. To support it, allow the left arm to hug your body and rest your right elbow on top of the arm. If you have a cold or sinus infection, skip this technique.

ADVANCED ENERGETIC NADI SHODHANA

Alternate Nostril Breathing

TIME: 15 minutes

BENEFITS: Improved Focus, Energy, Mental Clarity, Strengthened Intuition

This advanced version of Energetic Nadi Shodhana (page 96) creates more space for your mind to clear, and your focus and intuition to strengthen, with longer kumbhaka, or breath retention (page 28), after your inhalation. This longer hold will enhance the brahmana energetic effect (page 6) that this practice offers.

1. Set a timer for 15 minutes.

2. In a comfortable seated posture with your spine erect, close your eyes and relax your body.

3. Establish an even breathing rhythm (Sama Vritti, page 52), inhaling for a count of six and exhaling for a count of six. Continue for 2 minutes.

   ☀ Simplified: Inhale (6), Exhale (6)

4. Extend your breathing to an eight-count even breath. Continue for 2 minutes.

   ☀ Simplified: Inhale (8), Exhale (8)

5. Bring your right hand into Vishnu Mudra (page 38). Block your right nostril with your thumb and inhale through your left nostril for a count of eight.

6. Close both nostrils and hold the breath in for a count of eight, while engaging Jalandhara Bandha (page 14).

7. Release your right nostril (keeping the left blocked) and exhale for a count of eight.

8. Keeping the right nostril open, inhale for a count of eight.

9. Close both nostrils and hold the breath in for a count of eight, engaging Jalandhara Bandha.

10. Release your left nostril (keeping the right blocked) and exhale for a count of eight.

   ✳ Simplified:
   • Inhale Left (8), Hold In (8), Exhale Right (8)
   • Inhale Right (8), Hold In (8), Exhale Left (8)

11. Repeat steps 5 through 10 for 6 minutes (for a minimum of six rounds).

12. Release the mudra, breathe through both nostrils, and rest for 1 to 2 minutes with your eyes closed, aware of any sensations, especially at the center of your brain.

13. Journal your experience, noting any peculiar sensations, progress, and challenges.

TIPS: If one nostril is either partially or completely blocked, loosen the closed nostril slightly while still imagining air flowing through the opened nostril. Sometimes the right arm can get fatigued during this practice. To support it, allow the left arm to hug your body and rest your right elbow on top of the arm. If you have a cold or sinus infection, skip this technique.

BALANCING UJJAYI KRAMA PRANAYAMA

Segmented Ocean Breathing

TIME: 12 minutes

BENEFITS: Calming, Balance, Improved Focus, Improved Circulation

This advanced pranayama blends the benefits of both Balancing Ujjayi Pranayama (page 78) and Balancing Krama Pranayama (page 98) techniques. The sound and pauses of the breath powerfully calm a restless mind and create the conditions for lasting calm and peace.

1. In a comfortable seated posture with your spine erect, close your eyes and relax your body.

    ❋ Employ Gyan Mudra (page 39) or Chin Mudra (page 40) if you'd like.

2. Bring your awareness to your natural breathing rhythm for 10 breaths, noting the current quality of your breath.

3. Feel the sensation of your breath at the back of your throat and constrict the glottis, or back of the throat, slightly to make a soft hissing or ocean-like sound as you inhale and exhale.

4. Keeping the breath audible, inhale for a count of eight and exhale for a count of eight for 10 rounds.

    ❋ Noting the capacity of your breath, begin to identify where the halfway points are during your inhalations and exhalations.

5. Breathing audibly, inhale to 50 percent of your breath capacity (four counts) and pause the breath for four counts. Inhale the remaining 50 percent of your breath (four counts) and pause with the breath held in for four counts.

6. Breathing audibly, exhale 50 percent of your breath capacity (four counts) and pause the breath for four counts. Exhale the remaining 50 percent of your breath (four counts) and pause with the breath held out for four counts.

7. Repeat steps 4 through 6 for 10 breaths.

☀ Simplified:
   • Inhale 50 percent (4), Pause (4), Inhale 50 percent (4), Pause (4)
   • Exhale 50 percent (4), Pause (4), Exhale 50 percent (4), Pause (4)

8. Allow the breath to come to an effortless state and pay attention to any sensations, noticing a calmer and stiller mind.

9. Journal your experience, noting any peculiar sensations, progress, and challenges.

TIP: It can be easy to run out of breath or to feel fatigue during this practice. If you find yourself straining at any point, take a break and return to the practice when your system has calmed.

CALMING UJJAYI KRAMA PRANAYAMA

Segmented Ocean Breathing

TIME: 12 minutes

BENEFITS: Calming, Improved Focus, Improved Circulation

Blending Calming Krama Pranayama (page 100) and Calming Ujjayi Pranayama (page 58) techniques while focusing on longer kumbhaka, or breath retention (page 28), during the exhalation strengthens the langhana effect (page 6) of these practices. Allow this technique to ground your mind, bringing you into a calmer and more peaceful state.

1. In a comfortable seated posture with your spine erect, close your eyes and relax your body.

    ✳ Employ Chin Mudra (page 40) if you'd like.

2. Bring your awareness to your natural breathing rhythm for 10 breaths, noting the current quality of your breath.

3. Feel the sensation of your breath at the back of your throat and constrict the glottis, or back of your throat, slightly to make a soft hissing or ocean-like sound as you inhale and exhale.

4. Keeping the breath audible, inhale for a count of eight and exhale for a count of eight for 10 rounds.

    ✳ Noting the capacity of your breath, identify where the halfway points are during your inhalations and exhalations.

5. Inhale a full eight-count breath with no retention.

6. Exhale to 50 percent of your breath capacity (four counts) and pause the breath for four counts. Exhale the remaining 50 percent of your breath (four counts) and pause with the breath held out for four counts.

7. Repeat steps 5 and 6 for 10 breaths.

   ✳ Simplified:
   - Inhale (8)
   - Exhale 50 percent (4), Pause (4), Exhale 50 percent (4), Pause (4)

8. Allow the breath to come to an effortless state and pay attention to any sensations, noticing a calmer and stiller mind.

9. Journal your experience, noting any peculiar sensations, progress, and challenges.

   TIP: An added component to this practice is to imagine your thoughts dissolving during the pauses. Your mind may be moving immediately afterward, but you'll be training your thoughts to become still.

ENERGIZING UJJAYI KRAMA PRANAYAMA

Segmented Ocean Breathing

TIME: 12 minutes
BENEFITS: Energy, Improved Focus

As you focus on pausing the breath intermittently during the inhalation, this variation of Krama Pranayama has a brahmana, or energizing energetic effect (page 6). This is a great technique to practice when you're feeling sluggish, lethargic, or depressed.

1. In a comfortable seated posture with your spine erect, close your eyes and relax your body.

   ✳ If you'd like to enhance the energizing effect, employ Gyan Mudra (page 39).

2. Bring your awareness to your natural breathing rhythm for 10 breaths, noting the current quality of your breath.

3. Feel the sensation of your breath at the back of your throat and constrict the glottis, or back of the throat, slightly to make a soft hissing or ocean-like sound as you inhale and exhale.

4. Keeping the breath audible, inhale for a count of eight and exhale for a count of eight for 10 rounds.

   ✳ Noting the capacity of your breath, identify where the halfway points are during your inhalations and exhalations.

5. Inhale to 50 percent of your breath capacity (four counts) and pause the breath for four counts. Inhale the remaining 50 percent of your breath (four counts) and pause with the breath held in for four counts.

6. Exhale a complete eight-count breath with no holds.

7. Repeat steps 5 and 6 for 10 breaths.

   ✳ Simplified:
   • Inhale 50 percent (4), Pause (4), Inhale 50 percent (4), Pause (4)
   • Exhale (8)

8. Allow the breath to come to an effortless state and pay attention to any sensations, noticing a calmer and stiller mind.

9. Journal your experience, noting any peculiar sensations, progress, and challenges.

   TIP: Be careful not to hold the breath longer than prescribed, as doing so is not sustainable and can cause you to lose your breath over time. Even a short pause is effective during this technique.

ENERGIZING KAPALABHATI
Shining Skull Breath

TIME: 12 minutes
BENEFITS: Mental Clarity, Detoxification, Improved Focus, Energy

This version of Kapalabhati (page 66) focuses on endurance with the practice and kumbhaka (page 28) repeatedly after the set of forced exhalations. The goal is to keep a consistent pace during the quick breathing and then to find stillness during the breath retention. This helps pull prana inward and upward, uplifting your consciousness.

1. In a comfortable seated posture with your spine erect, close your eyes and relax your body.

   ✳ If you'd like to enhance the energizing effect, employ Gyan Mudra (page 39).

2. Bring your awareness to your abdomen and feel your breath moving there for 1 minute.

3. Set a timer for 3 minutes.

4. Take a deep breath in through your nostrils, feel your abdomen expand, and then quickly and sharply exhale through both nostrils, feeling your navel pull back toward your spine. Allow the inhalation to expand in the abdomen quickly but passively (like a balloon filling) and quickly exhale through both nostrils again, feeling the abdomen snap back.

   ✳ The physical engagement of this technique is similar to blowing out a candle, but with your mouth closed—actively exhaling and passively inhaling through your nostrils.

❋ Note that the movement of your body is isolated to the abdomen. Attempting this technique breathing in your chest will lead to dizziness.

5. Repeat step 4 for 3 minutes straight without stopping.

6. After the final forced exhalation, inhale to fill your body, engage Jalandhara Bandha (page 14), and focus on light in your brain. Retain the breath until just beyond the point of comfort and then exhale slowly and with control.

7. Inhale immediately and hold the breath in again until just beyond the point of comfort and then exhale slowly and with control.

8. Repeat step 7 once more.

9. Relax and feel your breath adjust. Sit quietly for 3 minutes and notice the sensations of the practice. You might sense light in your brain, warmth in your abdomen, and spaciousness in your lungs.

10. Journal your experience, noting any peculiar sensations, progress, and challenges.

TIPS: Practice this technique at least 2 hours after eating. If you are pregnant, currently experiencing a heavy menstrual cycle, or have unregulated high blood pressure, you may want to skip this technique.

CALMING KAPALABHATI
Shining Skull Breath

TIME: 12 minutes

BENEFITS: Mental Clarity, Detoxification, Improved Focus, Calm

Calming Kapalabhati emphasizes long kumbhaka, or breath retention (page 28), after exhalation, including a forward fold. This combination grounds the clarifying effects of Kapalabhati (page 66) with the calming of your nervous system, leaving you calm, clear, and collected.

1. In a comfortable seated posture with your spine erect, close your eyes and relax your body. Though any seated posture is good for this practice, I recommend sitting in *Virasana* (page 36), also known as Hero's pose, for this technique, as you'll be better able to fold forward later on.

   ✳ If you'd like to encourage the grounding effect, employ Chin Mudra (page 40).

2. Bring your awareness to your abdomen and feel your breath moving there for 1 minute.

3. Set a timer for 3 minutes.

4. Take a deep breath in through your nostrils, feel your abdomen expand, and then quickly and sharply exhale through both nostrils, feeling your navel pull back toward your spine. Allow the inhalation to expand in the abdomen quickly but passively (like a balloon filling) and quickly exhale through both nostrils again, feeling the abdomen snap back.

✳ The physical engagement of this technique is similar to blowing out a candle, but with your mouth closed—actively exhaling and passively inhaling through your nostrils.

✳ Note that the movement of your body is isolated to the abdomen. Breathing in your chest for this technique will lead to dizziness.

5. Repeat step 4 for 3 minutes.

6. After the final forced exhalation, take a deep breath in, and without holding the breath in, exhale slowly and fold forward, bringing your forehead toward the ground. Hold the breath out until just beyond the point of comfort.

7. As you inhale, sit up to a tall spine and then immediately exhale slowly and fold forward again, holding the breath out until just beyond the point of comfort.

8. Repeat step 7 once more.

9. Stay in the forward fold as you inhale, breathing calmly for 1 minute.

10. With an inhalation, sit up tall and notice any sensations for 3 minutes. You might sense light in your brain, warmth in your abdomen, and spaciousness in your lungs.

11. Journal your experience, noting any peculiar sensations, progress, and challenges.

TIPS: Practice this technique at least 2 hours after eating. If you are pregnant, currently experiencing a heavy menstrual cycle, or have unregulated high blood pressure, you may want to skip this technique.

ADVANCED BHASTRIKA PRANAYAMA

Bellows Breath

TIME: 10 minutes

BENEFITS: Improved Digestion, Energy, Warmth

Once you've practiced the beginner version of Bhastrika Pranayama (page 88), you can advance to a longer and steadier version of the practice. This stoking of the digestive fire helps energize your navel chakra while simultaneously creating light in your mind.

1. In a comfortable seated posture with your spine erect, close your eyes and relax your body.

   ✳ If you'd like to enhance the energizing effect, employ Gyan Mudra (page 39).

2. Bring your awareness to your abdomen and feel your breath moving there for 1 minute.

3. Set a timer for 3 minutes.

4. Take a deep breath in through your nostrils, feeling your belly fill and expand forward.

5. Exhale powerfully through your nostrils, feeling your belly empty and your navel contract back toward your spine.

6. Repeat steps 4 and 5 for 3 minutes at a moderate pace.

   ✳ If you're able to, you can pick up the pace, but slow down if you start to feel dizzy.

   ✳ Be mindful to keep the spine tall and as still as possible the entire time, especially in your lower back.

7. Release the technique and sit tall, noticing any sensations, for 3 minutes. Gently allow the eyes to open.

8. Journal your experience, noting any peculiar sensations, progress, and challenges.

TIPS: Though you may feel energized, take the time to sit with the effects of the technique before moving on with your day. This helps settle and stabilize your energy. Practice this technique at least 2 hours after eating. If you are pregnant, currently experiencing a heavy menstrual cycle, or have unregulated high blood pressure, you may want to skip this technique.

ADVANCED SHEETALI ANULOMA PRANAYAMA

Cooling Alternate Nostril Breathing

TIME: 10 minutes

BENEFITS: Stress Relief, Cooling, Balance

Blending Sheetali Pranayama (page 70) and Nadi Shodhana, this practice will enhance the langhana effect (page 6) by adding a kumbhaka (page 28) after exhalation. The level of focus required for this practice helps pull your mind out of restless cycles and calms your nervous system.

1. In a comfortable seated posture with your spine erect, close your eyes and relax your body. Bring your right hand into Vishnu Mudra (page 38) for the alternate nostril breathing portion of this practice.

2. Establish an even six-count breathing rhythm for five breaths.

3. Stick your tongue out of your mouth and curl the sides up and inward to make a tube.

4. Inhale for six counts through the tube, feeling the cool sensation on the tongue, saliva, mouth, and throat.

5. Unroll your tongue. Block your right nostril with your thumb and exhale for six counts through your left nostril.

6. Hold your breath out for six counts.

7. Roll your tongue again and inhale for six counts through the tube.

8. Unroll your tongue. Block your left nostril with your ring finger and exhale for six counts through your right nostril.

9. Hold your breath out for six counts.

   ✳ Simplified: Inhale (6), Exhale Left (6), Hold Out (6), Inhale (6), Exhale Right (6), Hold Out (6)

10. Repeat steps 3 through 9 for 7 minutes.

11. Release the technique and feel the cooling, calming, and balancing sensations in your body and mind.

12. Journal your experience, noting any peculiar sensations, progress, and challenges.

TIPS: If you're unable to roll the tongue into a tube, you can do this same technique with the mouth in the position of Sheetkari Pranayama (page 72).

ANULOMA PRANAYAMA

TIME: 6 minutes
BENEFITS: Balance, Mental Clarity, Detoxification, Improved
Focus, Strengthened Intuition

This alternate nostril pranayama focuses on clear inhalation
through both nostrils with a sharp and quick exhalation in
alternating nostrils. This helps cleanse and purify the nadis,
increasing the flow of prana throughout your body.

1. In a comfortable seated posture with your spine erect, close
   your eyes and relax your body.

2. Bring your awareness to your natural breathing rhythm for
   10 breaths, noting the current quality of your breath.

3. Bring your right hand into Vishnu Mudra (page 38).

4. Take a slow and deep inhalation through both nostrils, feeling
   the coolness of your breath in the nasal passages.

5. Block your right nostril and exhale sharply through your left
   nostril, feeling your navel contract toward your spine.

6. Open both nostrils and inhale deeply through both nostrils.

7. Repeat steps 5 and 6 for three total rounds.

8. Breathe softly and fully through both nostrils for three
   breaths.

9. Inhale deeply through both nostrils.

10. Block your left nostril and exhale sharply through your right
    nostril, again feeling your navel pull back toward your spine.

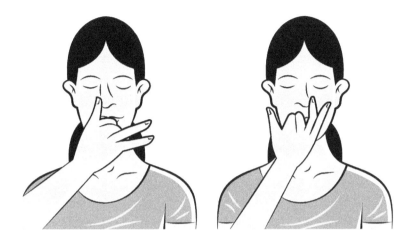

11. Open both nostrils and inhale deeply through both nostrils.

12. Repeat steps 10 and 11 for three total rounds.

13. Breathe softly and fully through both nostrils for three breaths.

14. Release the technique and pay attention to any sensations, especially in your head.

15. Journal your experience, noting any peculiar sensations, progress, and challenges.

TIPS: Have tissues nearby to wipe your nose after the practice. If one nostril is either partially or completely blocked, loosen the closed nostril slightly while still imagining air flowing through the opened nostril. If you have a cold or sinus infection, skip this practice.

PRATILOMA PRANAYAMA

Inverted Alternate Nostril Breathing

TIME: 10 minutes

BENEFITS: Calming, Stress Relief, Mental Clarity, Improved Focus

Also known as Inverted Anuloma Pranayama, *Pratiloma* focuses on alternating nostrils while inhaling, and slowing down the exhalation, giving this technique more of a langhana, or calming energetic effect (page 6).

1. Set a timer for 10 minutes.

2. In a comfortable seated posture with your spine erect, close your eyes and relax your body.

3. Bring your awareness to your natural breathing rhythm for 10 breaths, noting the current quality of your breath.

4. Bring your right hand into Vishnu Mudra (page 38).

5. Blocking your right nostril, take a slow, deep inhalation through your left nostril.

6. Open both nostrils and exhale slowly through both nostrils, ideally longer than the inhalation. You can count the breath if that's helpful.

7. Block your left nostril and take a slow, deep inhalation through your right nostril.

8. Open both nostrils and exhale slowly through both nostrils, extending your exhalation.

9. Repeat steps 5 through 8 for 7 minutes.

10. Release the technique and pay attention to any sensations, especially in your head.

11. Journal your experience, noting any peculiar sensations, progress, and challenges.

TIPS: If one nostril is either partially or completely blocked, loosen the closed nostril slightly while still imagining air flowing through the opened nostril. If you have a cold or sinus infection, skip this practice.

CHANDRA BHEDANA PRANAYAMA

Moon-Piercing Breath

TIME: 5 to 7 minutes

BENEFITS: Cooling, Calming, Improved Focus

Chandra Bhedana is a powerful calming pranayama combining alternate nostril breathing with kumbhaka (page 28). Though a brief practice, its activation of the ida nadi (page 10) induces a strong langhana energetic effect (page 6).

1. In a comfortable seated posture with your spine erect, close your eyes and relax your body.

2. Bring your awareness to your natural breathing rhythm for 10 breaths, noting the current quality of your breath.

3. Bring your right hand into Vishnu Mudra (page 38).

4. Blocking your right nostril, inhale slowly and deeply through your left nostril.

5. Block your left nostril and exhale slowly and completely through your right nostril.

6. Block both nostrils and hold your breath out for as long as is comfortable.

7. Repeat steps 4 through 6 for five rounds.

   ❋ If you need to, relax and breathe normally between rounds, concentrating on light in your brain.

8. Sit and notice any sensations for 1 to 2 minutes.

9. Journal your experience, noting any peculiar sensations, progress, and challenges.

TIPS: If this technique causes any anxiety in your system, save it for another day. If you have unregulated high blood pressure, you can skip this technique. Don't practice this technique and *Surya Bhedana Pranayama* (page 134) on the same day.

SURYA BHEDANA PRANAYAMA

Sun-Piercing Breath

TIME: 10 to 12 minutes

BENEFITS: Energy, Mental Clarity, Improved Focus

This energizing pranayama technique helps build vitality in your body and mind, as well as clear any fogginess. Surya Bhedana is a great graduation from Advanced Energetic Nadi Shodhana (page 112).

1. In a comfortable seated posture with your spine erect, close your eyes and relax your body.

2. Bring your awareness to your natural breathing rhythm for 10 breaths, noting the current quality of your breath.

3. Bring your right hand into Vishnu Mudra (page 38).

4. Blocking your left nostril, inhale slowly and deeply through your right nostril.

5. Block both nostrils and hold the breath in, engaging both Jalandhara Bandha (page 14) and Mula Bandha (page 14). Hold for as long as you can, visualizing light in your brain.

6. Release the bandhas, keep the right nostril blocked, and exhale slowly through your left nostril.

7. Repeat steps 4 through 6 for 10 rounds.

※ If you need to, relax and breathe normally between rounds, continuing to concentrate on light in your brain.

8. Sit and notice sensations for 1 to 2 minutes.

9. Journal your experience, noting any peculiar sensations, progress, and challenges.

TIPS: If this technique causes any anxiety in your system, save it for another day. If you have unregulated high blood pressure, you can skip this technique. Don't practice this technique and Chandra Bhedana Pranayama (page 132) on the same day.

MOORCHA PRANAYAMA
Swooning Breath

TIME: 8 to 10 minutes

BENEFITS: Mental Clarity, Improved Focus, Strengthened Intuition

Moorcha Pranayama is specifically designed to strengthen your intuition; this technique helps make the unconscious conscious. Though simple in explanation, this technique should be practiced only after comfort and mastery of other practices involving kumbhaka (page 28) has been achieved. Its ability to still the mind makes it a great preparatory step for deeper meditation.

1. In a comfortable seated posture with your spine erect, close your eyes and relax your body. Place your hands palm down on your knees. No mudra should be used for this technique.

2. Bring your awareness to your natural breathing rhythm for 10 breaths, noting the current quality of your breath.

3. Closing your eyes, inhale slowly and deeply through your nostrils.

4. Hold your breath in, engaging Jalandhara Bandha (page 14) and focusing on the space between your eyebrows. Keep holding your breath in for even longer than is comfortable.

5. Keeping your eyes closed, release Jalandhara Bandha, raise your chin (see image), and exhale slowly and with strong control.

6. Breathe normally, focusing on the space between your eyebrows for 1 to 2 minutes.

7. Repeat steps 3 through 6 for five total rounds.

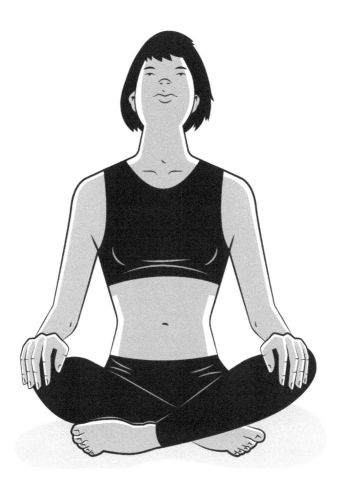

8. Sit and notice any sensations for 1 to 2 minutes.

9. Journal your experience, noting any peculiar sensations, progress, and challenges.

TIPS: This technique is recommended for practitioners who have a strong capacity for extended kumbhaka, or breath retention (page 28). If you notice lightheadedness while practicing, save this technique for another day. If you have unregulated high blood pressure, skip this practice.

six

PRANAYAMA IN PRACTICE

In this chapter, we'll weave individual pranayama techniques together into intentional sequences. The effects of these techniques can be enhanced when combined, and some can be warm-ups for others. For example, if your nostrils are partially blocked and Nadi Shodhana is difficult, you could practice Kapalabhati (page 66) beforehand to clear the nasal passages.

These sequences are labeled with their level of difficulty, so as with the individual practices, start at the beginning and build your energetic competency before you progress. There is no rush to master any of the practices given here, and some techniques or sequences may be appropriate for you only some of the time. Trust your own inner guidance.

NATURAL BALANCE

TIME: 12 minutes
DIFFICULTY LEVEL: Beginner
BENEFITS: Calming, Balance, Increased Lung Capacity

Natural Balance is a great practice to start regulating your breath and to consistently expand your lung capacity. You will also be creating the perfect lung capacity to build toward Sama Vritti (page 52) at the end of the sequence. If your breath is feeling shallow and stagnant, try this sequence out.

1. Set a timer for 12 minutes.

2. In a comfortable posture, sitting tall or lying down in Savasana (page 37), allow your eyes to close, and relax your whole body.

3. Begin with the Natural Breathing technique (page 44) and allow yourself to be effortless in your body. Shorten the duration of each stage of awareness to five breaths. Note the current capacity of your breath (shallow versus deep). Stay engaged with this technique for at least 2 minutes.

4. Continue on to the Expanded Breathing practice (page 46) for 2 minutes. The gentle expansion of your lung capacity will prepare you for the next stage of this sequence. Notice how your lung capacity actually grows from breath to breath.

5. Begin to balance out your breath with the Sama Vritti practice (page 52) with a six-count breath for at least 5 minutes. Having built to this technique with the Expanded Breathing practice, notice if it's easier for you to achieve an effortless six-count breath than it was when you practiced Sama Vritti alone.

※ Simplified: Inhale (6), Exhale (6)

6. Release all techniques and rest your awareness in the spaciousness of your body, particularly your lungs and chest. Notice how your breath may naturally rest at a fuller lung capacity. Return your awareness to this expanded capacity throughout your day.

7. Journal your experience, progress, and notable sensations.

TIP: This sequence can be lengthened or shortened easily, depending on how much time you have. It's safe to stay in each stage for as long or short as you need; just be sure to give a fair amount of time to Sama Vritti at the end.

A CLEAR DAY

TIME: 12 minutes
DIFFICULTY LEVEL: Beginner
BENEFITS: Energy, Balance, Mental Clarity, Improved
Focus, Warmth

Start your day with this quick sequence to get your mind clear, balanced, and energized to tackle whatever awaits you. The systematic building of this sequence creates strong clarity, especially within your nostrils, aiding in the practice of Balancing Nadi Shodhana (page 62) later in this sequence.

1. In a comfortable seated posture with your spine erect, close your eyes and relax your body.

   ☀ If you'd like to enhance the energizing effect, employ Gyan Mudra (page 39) for the first two steps of this sequence.

2. Begin with the Natural Breathing technique (page 44) and really allow yourself to be effortless in your body. Shorten the duration of each stage of awareness to five breaths. When you get to the awareness of your breath in your abdomen, stay with the sensation for at least 10 breaths, as this awareness will help prepare you for the next step. Continue this practice for at least 2 minutes.

3. Next, move on to Kapalabhati (page 66) and complete three total rounds of 27 breaths each. As you practice this technique, see light building in the center of your brain as if you're charging light at that point and clearing your mind.

4. Rest from the final round of Kapalabhati for 1 minute, continuing to see the light in your brain.

5. Lastly, practice Balancing Nadi Shodhana, switching your hand mudra into Vishnu Mudra (page 38). Practice for 5 minutes with a six-count breath.

   ❋ Simplified: Inhale Left (6), Exhale Right (6), Inhale Right (6), Exhale Left (6)

6. Release all the techniques and feel your breath moving smoothly through both nostrils. Slowly allow your eyes to open, noticing the sensation.

7. Journal your experience, progress, and notable sensations.

   TIPS: You can raise the level of this technique by using the intermediate version of Kapalabhati (page 84) and the intermediate or advanced versions of Balancing Nadi Shodhana (pages 92 and 108).

EXPANSIVE CALM

TIME: 10 minutes
DIFFICULTY LEVEL: Beginner
BENEFITS: Calming, Stress Relief, Improved Circulation,
Increased Lung Capacity

Increase your lung capacity and ground your nervous system
with this sequence that combines Dirgha Pranayama
(page 56) and Calming Ujjayi Pranayama (page 58).
Expansive Calm is a great practice for when you're feeling
constricted and need to create more internal space for
acceptance and compassion.

1. Set a timer for 10 minutes.

2. In a comfortable seated posture with your spine erect, close
   your eyes and relax your body.

   ※ If you'd like to enhance the grounding and calming effect of
   this sequence, employ Chin Mudra (page 40).

3. Employ Dirgha Pranayama, establishing a smooth three-part
   breath for 3 minutes.

   ※ Simplified:
   • Inhale: Abdomen > Rib Cage > Collarbones
   • Exhale: Collarbones > Rib Cage > Abdomen

4. Keeping Dirgha Pranayama engaged, include Calming Ujjayi Pranayama by first constricting the glottis, or back of the throat, slightly to make a soft hissing or ocean-like sound as you inhale and exhale. Continue for 1 minute.

    ✳ If your throat feels strained as you inhale, make your breath audible on exhalation only. As your throat adjusts to Ujjayi, it will become easier to make audible on the inhalation.

5. With this three-part audible breath, begin to lengthen and slow your exhalation to make it twice as long as your inhalation. I suggest inhaling for a count of four and exhaling for a count of eight, again all while maintaining Dirgha Pranayama. Continue for 5 minutes.

    ✳ Simplified: Inhale (4); Exhale (8)

6. Release all the techniques and focus on your own internal stillness, noting any additional sensations. Take your time as you come back.

7. Journal your experience, progress, and notable sensations.

TIPS: Take more time in the individual Dirgha Pranayama practice if you're having a hard time achieving the three-part breath. You can also use internal imagery, imagining that your breath is moving up your spine as you inhale and moving down your spine as you exhale.

AWAKEN INTUITION

TIME: 8 to 10 minutes
DIFFICULTY LEVEL: Beginner
BENEFITS: Energy, Mental Clarity, Improved Focus, Strengthened Intuition, Warmth

Simulate your third eye center with this clarifying and energizing pranayama sequence. If you find yourself unable to decide between two or more plans of action, try this practice to still your restless thoughts and give yourself greater perspective.

1. In a comfortable seated posture with your spine erect, close your eyes and relax your body.

   ✳ If you'd like to enhance the energizing effect, employ Gyan Mudra (page 39) for the centering and Kapalabhati (page 66) portions of this sequence.

2. Bring your awareness to your natural breathing rhythm of your abdomen for a few rounds of breath.

3. Employ Kapalabhati and complete three total rounds of 27 breaths each. As you practice this technique, see light building in the center of your brain as if you're charging light at that point and clearing your mind.

4. Rest from the final round of Kapalabhati for 1 minute, continuing to see the light in your brain.

5. Set a timer for 3 minutes.

6. Next, employ 3 minutes of Bhramari Pranayama (page 68), moving your index fingers to the triangle flaps in front of your ear canals (the tragi).

  ✳ Because you'll be vibrating noise to the center of your brain, set your timer volume higher so you know when to release the practice.

7. Release all the techniques and bring your hands to rest on your knees. Take slow deep breaths, being aware of sensation and quiet in your mind. Stay as long as you need to.

8. Journal your experience, progress, and notable sensations.

TIP: You can raise the level of this technique by employing Intermediate Kapalabhati (page 84).

DEEP STILLNESS

TIME: 7 minutes
DIFFICULTY LEVEL: Beginner
BENEFITS: Calming, Stress Relief, Mental Clarity, Improved
Focus, Increased Lung Capacity

Take your Bhramari Pranayama (page 68) practice to a
new level by extending the breath. The bigger inhalations
will give you the endurance to last longer with each buzzing
exhalation, creating a calmer and quieter mind. Practice
this sequence to tap in to the awareness of deeper wisdom
within you.

1. In a comfortable seated posture with your spine erect, close
   your eyes and relax your body.

   ✳ If you'd like to enhance the grounding and calming effect of
     this sequence, employ Chin Mudra (page 40) during steps
     2 through 4.

2. Bring your awareness to your natural breathing rhythm for a
   few rounds of breath.

3. Continue on to the Expanded Breathing practice (page 46)
   for 2 minutes. The gentle expansion of your lung capacity will
   prepare you for the next stage of this sequence. Notice how
   your lung capacity actually grows from breath to breath.

4. Set a timer for 3 minutes.

5. Keeping your breath expanded, practice Bhramari Pranayama for 3 minutes, moving your index fingers to the triangle flaps in front of your ear canals (the tragi).

   ☀ With each inhalation, allow your lungs to again fill to capacity. This will help you last longer with each hum of Bhramari Pranayama.

   ☀ Because you'll be vibrating noise to the center of your brain, set your timer volume higher so you know when to release the practice.

6. Release all the techniques and bring your hands to rest on your knees. Take slow, deep breaths, paying attention to any sensations and the quiet in your mind. Stay as long as you need to.

7. Journal your experience, progress, and notable sensations.

   TIP: If you you have the endurance, you can extend your Bhramari practice to up to 5 minutes.

STRONG BEAST

TIME: 6 to 8 minutes
DIFFICULTY LEVEL: Beginner
BENEFITS: Stress Relief, Energy, Detoxification, Toning

Build up your "roar" with this Strong Beast sequence. Blending Dirgha Pranayama (page 56) and Simhasana Pranayama (page 60), the sequence will clear out your lungs, releasing more toxins and tension with every big exhalation. Feeling stressed and agitated? On the verge of yelling at someone? Sit and practice this sequence instead.

1. In a comfortable seated posture with your spine erect, close your eyes and relax your body.

   ✳ If you'd like to enhance the energizing effect, employ Gyan Mudra (page 39) for the Dirgha Pranayama portion of this sequence.

2. Bring your awareness to your natural breathing rhythm for a few rounds of breath.

3. Employ Dirgha Pranayama, establishing a smooth three-part breath for 3 minutes.

   ✳ Simplified:
      • Inhale: Abdomen > Rib Cage > Collarbones
      • Exhale: Collarbones > Rib Cage > Abdomen

✳ This systematic breath will help you steady your mind and energy, directing prana intentionally versus allowing it to move around erratically.

4. As you move into the Simhasana portion of this sequence, you'll keep the three-part inhalation.

5. Turn your palms up on your knees and splay your fingers wide with your arms stretched out. Complete five rounds of the Simhasana Pranayama, again inhaling in three parts each time.

✳ Simplified:
  • Inhale: Abdomen > Rib Cage > Collarbones
  • Exhale: Lion's Breath

6. Rest and feel your body adjust, noting any sensations and your mental-emotional state.

7. Journal your experience, progress, and notable sensations.

TIP: Practice the steps for the exhalation for Simhasana individually to familiarize yourself with the sequence.

MOVING THE BLOCK

TIME: 12 to 15 minutes
DIFFICULTY LEVEL: Intermediate
BENEFITS: Balance, Mental Clarity, Improved Focus, Improved Digestion, Warmth

This sequence will help you move past mental stagnation and lethargy, enabling you to be more decisive and creative. If you find yourself stuck and unable to make decisions or if you're in cycles of procrastination, sit and practice this sequence.

1. In a comfortable seated posture with your spine erect, close your eyes and relax your body.

   ☀ If you'd like to enhance the energizing effect, employ Gyan Mudra (page 39) for the Ujjayi and Bhastrika portions of this sequence.

2. Bring your awareness to your natural breathing rhythm for a few rounds of breath.

3. Begin Balancing Ujjayi Pranayama (page 78) for an even six-count breath, constricting the back of your throat, or glottis, to make the soft ocean sound as you breathe. Continue this technique for 2 minutes.

   ☀ Become aware of the movement of your abdomen as you breathe.

4. Next, move through three 1-minute rounds of Bhastrika Pranayama (page 88). Feel warmth and sensation building in your abdomen, and your mind clearing with each breath.

5. Relax from Bhastrika for 1 minute, simply noticing sensation and your breath in your body.

6. Lastly, practice Balancing Nadi Shodhana (page 62), switching your hand mudra into Vishnu Mudra (page 38). Practice for 5 minutes with an even six-count breath.

   ☀ Simplified: Inhale Left (6), Exhale Right (6), Inhale Right (6), Exhale Left (6)

7. Release all the techniques and feel your breath moving smoothly through both nostrils. Slowly allow your eyes to open, noticing any sensations.

8. Journal your experience, progress, and notable sensations.

TIPS: To raise the level of this sequence, try extending your Balancing Ujjayi Pranayama to an 8- or 10-count breathing rhythm.

BIG BALANCE

TIME: 10 minutes

DIFFICULTY LEVEL: Intermediate

BENEFITS: Calming, Stress Relief, Balance, Increased Lung Capacity

Build toward greater breath control as you systematically increase the lengths of your inhalations and exhalations with this Big Balance pranayama sequence. Starting small and working your way toward bigger breaths will help you cultivate a greater natural breathing capacity, giving you more oxygen in your bloodstream while keeping your nervous system grounded.

1. Set a timer for 10 minutes.

2. In a comfortable seated posture with your spine erect, close your eyes and relax your body.

   ✳ If you'd like, practice either Gyan Mudra (page 39) or Chin Mudra (page 40) with this sequence.

3. Bring your awareness to your natural breathing rhythm for a few breaths.

4. Begin with Balancing Ujjayi Pranayama (page 78), with a six-count even breath. Continue for at least 2 minutes, making sure that the even breath becomes less effortful over time.

   ✳ Simplified: Inhale (6), Exhale (6)

5. Keeping with the even breath, extend your breathing rhythm to eight counts by slowing down the intake of breath into your body on inhalation and slowing down the output of breath on exhalation. Continue for 3 minutes, establishing a sense of ease to this extended breathing rhythm before continuing.

✳ Simplified: Inhale (8), Exhale (8)

6. Lastly, extend your breathing rhythm to a 10-count even breath. Keep your breath at this capacity for 4 minutes, again establishing a sense of ease with the breath as you adjust to this greater capacity.

✳ Simplified: Inhale (10), Exhale (10)

7. Release all techniques and rest your awareness in any sensations in your body and mind.

8. Journal your experience, progress, and notable sensations.

TIPS: The Ujjayi constriction of the throat helps you gain control over the flow of air in and out of your body. Keep this audible breath engaged the entire time to help with that control. If you've mastered this sequence, you can continue to extend the breathing rhythm as your system feels ready.

CLEAR, CALM, COLLECTED

TIME: 15 minutes
DIFFICULTY LEVEL: Intermediate
BENEFITS: Balance, Mental Clarity, Detoxification, Improved Focus, Strengthened Intuition

Stoke energy at your third eye center with this clarifying sequence. Each technique woven into this sequence stimulates your intuitive center, giving you clearer access to knowledge and wisdom. This is a great practice when you need to make a tough decision or need higher wisdom.

1. In a comfortable seated posture with your spine erect, close your eyes and relax your body.

   ☀ If you'd like to enhance the energizing effect, employ Gyan Mudra (page 39) for the centering and Kapalabhati (page 66) portions of this sequence.

2. Bring your awareness to your natural breathing rhythm of your abdomen for a few rounds of breath.

3. Employ Kapalabhati, completing three rounds of 54 breaths each. As you practice this technique, see light building in the center of your brain as if you're charging light at that point and clearing your mind.

4. Rest from the final round of Kapalabhati for 1 minute, continuing to see light in your brain.

5. Set a timer for 3 minutes.

6. Practice Bhramari Pranayama (page 68) for 3 minutes, moving your index fingers to the triangle flaps in front of your ear canals (the tragi).

  ❋ Because you'll be vibrating noise to the center of your brain, set your timer volume higher so you know when to release the practice.

7. Rest from Bhramari for 1 minute, holding your awareness at the center of your brain.

8. Lastly, practice Balancing Nadi Shodhana (page 62), switching your hand mudra into Vishnu Mudra (page 38). Practice for 5 minutes with an even eight-count breath.

  ❋ Simplified: Inhale Left (8), Exhale Right (8), Inhale Right (8), Exhale Left (8)

9. Release all the techniques and feel your breath moving smoothly through both nostrils. Focus your awareness at the center of your brain, noticing any calmness or clarity.

10. Journal your experience, progress, and notable sensations.

TIPS: To raise the level of this sequence, try practicing Kapalabhati for 3 minutes straight instead for three 54-breath rounds.

STEADY AS YOU GO

TIME: 12 minutes
DIFFICULTY LEVEL: Intermediate
BENEFITS: Stress Relief, Balance, Mental Clarity, Improved Focus

This sequence pairs Dirgha Pranayama (page 56) with segmented breath, breaking your breathing rhythm into thirds with brief kumbhaka, or breath retention (page 28).

1. Set a timer for 10 minutes.

2. In a comfortable seated posture with your spine erect, close your eyes and relax your body.

   ✳ If you'd like to encourage the grounding effect of this sequence, employ Chin Mudra (page 40).

3. Bring your awareness to your natural breathing rhythm for a few rounds of breath.

4. Practice Dirgha Pranayama, establishing a smooth three-part breath for 3 minutes. Do your best to establish a nine-count, even breathing rhythm.

   ✳ Simplified:
      • Inhale: Abdomen > Rib Cage > Collarbones (9 counts)
      • Exhale: Collarbones > Rib Cage > Abdomen (9 counts)

5. Next, you'll insert two-count pauses at each third of your breath. Inhale for three counts (abdomen), pause for two counts, inhale for three counts (rib cage), pause for two counts, inhale for three counts (collarbones), and pause for two counts. Then exhale for three counts (collarbones), pause for two counts, exhale for three counts (rib cage), pause for two counts, exhale for three counts (abdomen), and pause for two counts. Repeat for 6 minutes.

☀ Simplified:
   • Inhale: Abdomen (3), Pause (2), Rib Cage (3), Pause (2), Collarbones (3), Pause (2)
   • Exhale: Collarbones (3), Pause (2), Rib Cage (3), Pause (2), Abdomen (3), Pause (2)

6. Release and allow your breath to adjust, resting into any sensations for 1 minute.

7. Journal your experience, progress, and notable sensations.

TIP: You may find yourself getting fatigued during this practice and in need of a normal breath. Allow yourself to stop when you feel anxious or uncomfortable, adjust, and then return to the practice when you can.

DIGESTIVE FIRE

TIME: 10 minutes
DIFFICULTY LEVEL: Intermediate
BENEFITS: Calming, Stress Relief, Mental Clarity, Improved
Digestion, Warmth

Stoke your digestive fire with this warming technique that
will help get your system moving. In this case, "digestion"
refers to both the body and the mind. When you're having a
hard time assimilating information from the world around
you, give this sequence a try.

1. In a comfortable seated posture with your spine erect, close
your eyes and relax your body.

    ☀ If you'd like to encourage the grounding effect of this
    sequence, employ Chin Mudra (page 40).

2. Bring your awareness to your natural breathing rhythm for a
few rounds of breath.

3. Notice your breath moving in your abdomen and establish
Diaphragmatic Breathing (page 48) for 3 minutes, softening
the effort in your abdomen and muscles of your pelvis. If you'd
like, you can place your dominant hand over your abdomen to
further ground your awareness.

4. Keeping your mind grounded in the movement of your abdomen, complete a 1-minute round of Bhastrika Pranayama (page 88), being sure that the movement of your body is isolated to the movement of your abdomen.

5. Return to Diaphragmatic Breathing for another 3 minutes, emphasizing the relaxation of the muscles in and around your abdomen and pelvis.

6. Relax the technique and breathe normally for a few moments before coming back.

7. Journal your experience, progress, and notable sensations.

TIP: If you need a little more from this practice, try adding one more 1-minute round of Bhastrika Pranayama, making sure to return to Diaphragmatic Breathing afterward.

CALM WINDS

TIME: 8 to 10 minutes
DIFFICULTY LEVEL: Advanced
BENEFITS: Balance, Mental Clarity, Improved Focus, Improved
Digestion, Warmth

Blending the forced breathing of Bhastrika Pranayama
(page 88) with the alternate nostril breathing of Anuloma
Pranayama (page 128) helps calm the restless fluctuations
of your mind by cleansing your nadis and bringing a clear
flow of prana to your system.

1. In a comfortable seated posture with your spine erect, close
   your eyes and relax your body.

2. Bring your awareness to your natural breathing rhythm
   for a few rounds of breath, noticing the movement of your
   abdomen.

3. Complete one 1-minute round of Bhastrika Pranayama.

4. Set a timer for 3 minutes.

5. Bring your right hand into Vishnu Mudra (page 38), preparing
   for alternate nostril breathing. For this next part, take a forced
   belly inhalation through both nostrils, block your right nostril,
   and exhale powerfully through your left nostril. Inhale forcefully through both nostrils, block your left nostril, and exhale
   powerfully through your right nostril. Repeat for 3 minutes.

✳ Simplified: Inhale Both, Exhale Left, Inhale Both, Exhale Right

✳ This blended technique should start slowly so that you can get used to the coordination of blocking and unblocking nostrils with forced breathing.

✳ If you start to feel dizzy, slow down or stop altogether and then return to the practice when you feel calmer.

6. Release all the techniques and feel your breath moving calmly through both nostrils and in your abdomen. Stay with the sensations for 2 to 3 minutes.

7. Journal your experience, progress, and notable sensations.

TIPS: Fatigue can happen with this sequence, especially in the early stages of practicing. If you need to rest, stop as needed, and then return to the practice when you feel ready. If you're feeling congested, try practicing Anuloma Pranayama separately beforehand.

STILL WATERS

TIME: 10 to 12 minutes
DIFFICULTY LEVEL: Advanced
BENEFITS: Calming, Stress Relief, Balance, Improved Focus

Still the restless states of mind that can keep you from calmness and stability with this advanced sequence. By inserting kumbhaka (page 28) during Balancing Nadi Shodhana (page 62), you create the conditions necessary for your mind to become as still as a calm lake.

1. In a comfortable seated posture with your spine erect, close your eyes and relax your body. Bring your awareness to your natural breathing rhythm for a few rounds of breath.

2. Set a timer for 2 minutes.

3. Place your index fingers over the triangle flaps in front of your ear canals (the tragi) and practice Bhramari Pranayama (page 68) for the full 2 minutes.

4. Release the technique and note the stillness developing in your mind.

5. Practice Balancing Nadi Shodhana, bringing your hand into Vishnu Mudra (page 38). Practice for 2 minutes with an even eight-count breath.

   ☀ Simplified: Inhale Left (8), Exhale Right (8), Inhale Right (8), Exhale Left (8)

6. Continuing Balancing Nadi Shodhana, you'll now insert short pauses at the halfway points of your breath.

   ☀ Blocking your right nostril, inhale to 50 percent for four counts, hold your breath for four counts, inhale the remaining 50 percent for four counts, and hold in for four counts.

✳ Release your right nostril and block your left nostril, then exhale 50 percent of your breath for four counts, hold the breath for four counts, exhale the remaining 50 percent for four counts, and hold out for four counts.

✳ Keep the nasal hold, inhale to 50 percent for four counts, hold your breath for four counts, inhale the remaining 50 percent, and hold in for four counts.

✳ Release your left nostril and block your right nostril, exhaling 50 percent of your breath for four counts, hold the breath for four counts, exhale remaining 50 percent for four counts, and hold out for four counts.

✳ Simplified:
- Inhale Left 50 percent (4), Hold (4), Inhale Left 50 percent (4), Hold (4)
- Exhale Right 50 percent (4), Hold (4), Exhale Right 50 percent (4), Hold (4)
- Inhale Right 50 percent (4), Hold (4), Inhale Right 50 percent (4), Hold (4)
- Exhale Left 50 percent (4), Hold (4), Exhale Left 50 percent (4), Hold (4)

7. Repeat step 6 for 5 minutes or for at least six rounds.

8. Release all the techniques and keep the breath calm and steady, noticing any sensations in your mind and body.

9. Journal your experience, progress, and notable sensations.

TIP: This technique takes a lot of breath control, so be gentle with yourself. If you need to take a break or shorten the practice, allow yourself to do so.

AWAKEN GREATNESS

TIME: 23 to 25 minutes
DIFFICULTY LEVEL: Advanced
BENEFITS: Balance, Energy, Mental Clarity, Improved Focus, Strengthened Intuition

This advanced pranayama sequence takes time and patience, pulling you out of your daily grind and asking you to rest into the internal stability within you. This sequence is a perfect preparation for deeper meditations or inner contemplations.

1. In a comfortable seated posture with your spine erect, close your eyes and relax your body.

2. Bring your awareness to your natural breathing rhythm for a few breaths, noticing the movement of your abdomen.

3. Set a timer for 3 minutes.

4. Practice Kapalabhati (page 66) for 3 minutes, building the sensation of light in your brain.

5. Rest for 1 minute, noticing light in your brain.

6. Set a timer for 4 minutes.

7. Bring your hand into Vishnu Mudra (page 38) and begin Pratiloma Pranayama (page 130) for 4 minutes.

8. Rest for 1 minute.

9. Lastly, practice Moorcha Pranayama (page 136) for five total rounds of breath, making sure to rest for at least 1 minute between each round.

10. Rest your awareness at the space between your eyebrows, breathing calmly for several minutes. Either come back to your day or move into a meditation practice.

11. Journal your experience, progress, and notable sensations.

TIPS: This is the longest of the sequences offered in this text, so make sure you're comfortably seated for this practice. It's okay to sit in a chair versus on the floor. It's also okay to use extra props to make yourself more comfortable. Refer to the posture options in chapter 2 (page 32).

BUILD YOUR OWN SEQUENCE!

Building your own pranayama sequence can be quite easy as you become more familiar with the individual techniques. Here are some questions to keep in mind as you're building your sequence:

1. What is your current practice level?

2. What is your current energetic state, and what energetic effect or benefits would you like to cultivate? See chapter 1 (page 6) for energetic effects.

3. How much time do you have?

4. What are your favorite pranayama techniques?

As you can imagine, if you want a beginner practice, you'll pick techniques only from chapter 3 (page 43). If you're building an intermediate or advanced practice, you still may use beginner techniques in your sequence. Blending techniques that have similar energetic effects is your next consideration. Do you want to be energized? Balanced? Calm? Look at the titles and benefits of different techniques and see which ones match best with what you are looking to achieve. Lastly, think about the complexity of the techniques. Generally, you'll want to start with simpler techniques and build your way toward ones that are more complex. For example, you may start any sequence with Natural Breathing (page 44), as it's the simplest technical technique offered here. From there, you could move on to Sama Vritti (page 52), and then onto Balancing Nadi Shodhana (page 62).

As you gain greater competency with the techniques offered in this book, you'll start to sense what feels right for combining techniques together. A good rule overall is to sequence no more than three or four techniques at one time. Often, less can be much more.

Resources

Books

Desikachar, T. K. V. *The Heart of Yoga: Developing a Personal Practice.* Rochester, VT: Inner Traditions International, 1995.
An easy read, this book is a great beginner's guide to yogic principles, including pranayama. It gives the reader a great understanding of how pranayama fits into the wider discipline of yoga.

Kraftsow, Gary. *Yoga for Wellness: Healing with the Timeless Teachings of Viniyoga.* New York: Penguin, 1999.
Though this book focuses on therapeutic yoga, the concepts around the energetic effects of practices, including pranayama, are explained in detail.

Mirsky, Karina Ayn, MA. *Make a Difference & Make a Living Teaching Yoga: The Secret to Transforming Lives While Supporting YourSelf.* Kalamazoo, MI: Yoga Mind Press, 2019.
Along with some variations on pranayama techniques, this book goes into detail about the energetic effects of practices.

Muktibodhananda, Swami. *Hatha Yoga Pradipika.* Bihar, India: Bihar School of Yoga, 1985.
As one of the core texts of hatha yoga, Hatha Yoga Pradipika *lists many pranayama techniques, including various variations.*

Websites

The Himalayan Institute: HimalayanInstitute.com
Great articles, videos, and audio on all things yoga.

Insight Timer: InsightTimer.com
A vast free library of audio practices. Search "Jerry Givens" to find my recorded practices.

Swami Jnaneshvara: SwamiJ.com
Amazing resource and commentary on all things classical yoga.

Yoga International: YogaInternational.com
Great articles, videos, and audio on all things yoga.

References

Bryant, Edwin F. *The Yoga Sūtras of Patañjali: A New Edition, Translation, and Commentary*. New York: North Point Press, 2009.

Clear, James. "How Long Does It Actually Take to Form a New Habit? (Backed by Science)." Accessed October 16, 2019. https://jamesclear.com/new-habit.

Core Walking. "Four Types of Breathing." Accessed October 16, 2019. https://corewalking.com/four-types-of-breathing/

Desikachar, T. K. V. *The Heart of Yoga: Developing a Personal Practice* (Rochester, VT: Inner Traditions International, 1995).

Gilbert, C. "Hyperventilation and the Body." Pub Med. Accessed October 16, 2019. https://www.ncbi.nlm.nih.gov/pubmed/10693382.

Gilbert, Christopher. "Better Chemistry Through Breathing: The Story of Carbon Dioxide and How It Can Go Wrong." Study Lib. Accessed October 16, 2019. https://studylib.net/doc/8718881/the-story-of-carbon-dioxide-and-how-it-can-go-wrong.

Healthline. "Bronchi." Accessed October 15, 2019. https://www.healthline.com/human-body-maps/bronchi#1.

Healthline. "Diaphragm Diagram." Accessed October 15, 2019. https://www.healthline.com/human-body-maps/diaphragm#diagram.

Healthline. "What You Should Know About Paradoxical Breathing." Accessed October 16, 2019. https://www.healthline.com/health/paradoxical-breathing#symptoms.

Kraftsow, Gary. *Yoga for Wellness: Healing with the Timeless Teachings of Viniyoga.* New York: Penguin Compass, 1999.

Mindmonia. "The 11 Best Mudras for Deeper Meditation." Accessed October 17, 2019. https://mindmonia.com/mudras.

Mirsky, Karina Ayn. *Sangha Yoga Advanced Teacher Training Manual: The Art & Science of Teaching Tantric Hatha Yoga.* Kalamazoo, MI: Sangha Yoga, 2013.

Muktibodhananada, Swami. *The Hatha Yoga Pradipika: Light on Hatha Yoga,* 3rd ed. Munger, Bihar, India: Yoga Publications Trust, 1998.

Power of Positivity. "Doctor Explains How to Relieve Anxiety Instantly Using Your Vagus Nerve." Accessed October 16, 2019. https://www.powerofpositivity.com/relieve-anxiety-vagus-nerve.

Stanford Health Care. "Turbinate Reduction." Accessed October 15, 2019. https://stanfordhealthcare.org/medical-treatments/n/nasal-surgery/types/turbinate-reduction.html.

Vivekananda, Dr. Rishi. *Practical Yoga Psychology*. Munger, Bihar, India: Yoga Publications Trust, 2005.

Index

Acknowledgments

The vast knowledge contained in this book would not have been possible if it weren't for the invaluable and continual support of my own teacher, Karina Ayn Mirsky, MA. Karina guided my first yoga class, and she continued to support me in the production of this book, spending hours hashing through techniques, variations, and deep wisdom around this sacred tradition. So much gratitude to you, Karina. May the work we do in this world never cease to illuminate others.

Deep gratitude to my best friend and sister in life, Sandy Huynh, MFT, who has been an anchor of emotional and psychological support during the writing of this book and for as long as I've known her. Here's to another great adventure!

Special thanks to my nearest and dearest dream team of supporters: Roseann Givens, Kenny Givens, Angelia Lane, Joe Somodi, Vanessa Kaul, Suzanne Roche, and Katherine Genis.

Lastly, I honor the unbroken lineage of my tradition, Sri Vidya, whose teachings on the science of yoga have been a life raft during the rough seas of my life. Gratitude to all the teachers who came before me.

About the Author

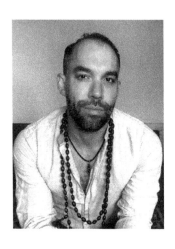

Jerry Givens is a yoga and meditation educator, retreat leader, writer, and life coach in the San Francisco Bay Area. He is a 500-hour certified teacher of Tantric Hatha Yoga & Meditation and has been teaching since 2008. He now leads yoga and meditation classes locally, frequent workshops and seminars, and annual retreats in Northern California. His life coaching is a blend of holistic yogic psychological interventions and the Internal Family Systems model of psychotherapy. As a writer, he has contributed to several online yoga publications and is also the author of three fantasy novels. Stay in touch with him at JerryGivens.net.

CPSIA information can be obtained
at www.ICGtesting.com
Printed in the USA
LVHW071740220222
711731LV00010B/315

9 781646 117390